Weight Loss for Women

The Ultimate Guide to Transform Your Body and Proven Strategies and Techniques to Achieve Your Health and Fitness Goals

Laura Trenaman

Table of Contents

Introduction 8

Chapter 1: Understanding Weight Loss for Women 12

1.1 The Science of Weight Loss 15

1.2 Differences in Male and Female Metabolism 20

1.3 Common Myths and Misconceptions 26

1.4 The Importance of Setting Realistic Goals 31

Chapter 2: Nutrition Essentials 35

2.1 Balanced Diet Fundamentals 42

2.2 Macronutrients: Proteins, Carbs, and Fats 46

2.3 Micronutrients: Vitamins and Minerals 50

2.4 Meal Planning and Preparation 54

2.5 Healthy and Delicious Recipes 58

Chapter 3: Effective Exercise Strategies 63

3.1 Cardio Workouts: Benefits and Types 68

3.2 Strength Training for Women 71

3.3 Flexibility and Mobility Exercises 75

3.5 Home Workouts vs. Gym Workouts 83

Chapter 4: Lifestyle and Behavioral Changes 87

4.1 Building Healthy Habits..90

4.2 Overcoming Emotional Eating 92

4.3 Stress Management Techniques 95

4.4 The Role of Sleep in Weight Loss 99

4.5 Staying Motivated and Consistent 102

Chapter 5: Understanding and Using Supplements..105

5.1 Overview of Popular Supplements 108

5.2 Benefits and Risks of Supplements 111

5.3 How to Choose the Right Supplements 114

5.4 Integrating Supplements into Your Routine 117

Chapter 6: Monitoring Progress and Adjusting Goals 121

6.1 Tracking Your Progress 124

6.2 Understanding Plateaus and How to Overcome Them 127

6.3 Adapting Your Plan for Continued Success 129

6.4 Celebrating Milestones and Achievements 133

Chapter 7: Long-Term Success and Maintenance 137

7.1 Transitioning from Weight Loss to Maintenance 139

7.2 Maintaining a Healthy Lifestyle 142

7.3 Dealing with Setbacks and Relapses 145

7.4 Building a Support System 149

7.5 The Journey to Lifelong Health and Fitness 151

Conclusion: 154

Introduction

Welcome to "Weight Loss for Women: The Ultimate Guide to Transform Your Body and Proven Strategies and Techniques to Achieve Your Health and Fitness Goals." This book is designed specifically for women who are ready to embark on a journey toward better health, enhanced fitness, and a more vibrant life. Whether you are looking to shed a few pounds, improve your overall well-being, or completely transform your body, this guide will provide you with the knowledge, tools, and motivation to succeed.

In a world overflowing with information about diet, exercise, and wellness, it can be challenging to navigate through the noise and find strategies that truly work. This book aims to cut through the confusion and deliver clear, evidence-based guidance tailored to the unique needs of women. Weight loss is not just about the number on the scale; it is about achieving a balance that promotes long-term health, self-confidence, and happiness.

Why Focus on Women?

Women face distinct physiological, hormonal, and psychological factors that influence their weight loss journey. From the impacts of menstrual cycles and menopause to the demands of pregnancy and motherhood, women's bodies are constantly changing. Understanding these dynamics is crucial for developing effective weight loss strategies that are both sustainable and compassionate.

What You Will Learn

This book covers a comprehensive range of topics, including:

- **Understanding Your Body**: Learn about the female anatomy, metabolism, and the role of hormones in weight management.
- **Nutrition Essentials**: Discover how to fuel your body with the right foods, understand portion sizes, and develop healthy eating habits that can be maintained for life.
- **Effective Workouts**: Find out which types of exercises are most effective for weight loss, strength building, and overall fitness. Whether you prefer cardio, strength training, yoga, or a combination of all three, you will find detailed plans to suit your lifestyle.
- **Mindset and Motivation**: Explore the psychological aspects of weight loss, including goal setting, overcoming mental barriers, and developing a positive self-image.
- **Lifestyle Changes**: Learn how to incorporate small but significant changes into your daily routine that will support your weight loss and health goals.
- **Expert Advice**: Gain insights from nutritionists, fitness trainers, and health professionals who specialize in women's health and fitness.

Our Approach

Our approach is holistic and compassionate. We believe that weight loss should not be about deprivation or extreme measures but about creating a healthy, balanced, and enjoyable lifestyle. This book encourages you to listen to your body, understand its needs, and make informed choices that empower you to achieve your goals.

Your Journey Starts Here

Embarking on a weight loss journey is a personal and empowering decision. This book is here to support you every step of the way, providing you with the tools and confidence to make lasting changes. Remember, the path to a healthier you is not a sprint but a marathon. It requires patience, perseverance, and self-love.

As you turn the pages, you will find practical advice, inspiring stories, and actionable steps that you can start implementing today. Get ready to transform your body, mind, and spirit, and embrace the incredible potential that lies within you.

Welcome to the beginning of your transformation. Let's start this journey together.

Chapter 1: Understanding Weight Loss for Women

Embarking on a weight loss journey requires a fundamental understanding of how your body works and what makes it unique. Women face distinct challenges and opportunities in their quest for a healthier body, and recognizing these differences is the first step toward effective and sustainable weight loss. In this chapter, we will explore the biological, hormonal, and psychological factors that play crucial roles in weight management for women.

The Biology of Weight Loss

To understand weight loss, it's essential to grasp the basics of metabolism. Metabolism is the process by which your body converts food into energy. It involves a series of chemical reactions that break down the calories from food and beverages into energy your body can use for daily activities and bodily functions.

- **Basal Metabolic Rate (BMR)**: This is the number of calories your body needs to maintain basic physiological functions such as breathing, circulation, and cell production while at rest. Women typically have a lower BMR compared to men due to differences in muscle mass and body composition. Increasing muscle mass through strength training can boost your BMR, helping you burn more calories even when at rest.
- **Total Daily Energy Expenditure (TDEE)**: Your TDEE is the total number of calories you burn in a day, including those burned through physical activity and digestion. Understanding your TDEE

can help you determine how many calories you need to consume to lose, maintain, or gain weight.

Hormonal Influences

Hormones play a significant role in weight management for women. They affect how your body stores and burns fat, your appetite, and even your mood. Key hormones that impact weight loss include:

- **Estrogen**: This hormone fluctuates throughout your menstrual cycle and can influence weight gain, especially around the hips and thighs. During menopause, estrogen levels decline, which can lead to an increase in abdominal fat.
- **Progesterone**: This hormone works in tandem with estrogen and can cause water retention and bloating, especially in the second half of the menstrual cycle.
- **Insulin**: Insulin regulates blood sugar levels and fat storage. Insulin resistance, a common issue among women with polycystic ovary syndrome (PCOS) and other conditions, can make weight loss more challenging.
- **Cortisol**: Known as the stress hormone, cortisol can lead to weight gain, particularly in the abdominal area, when levels are chronically elevated.

Understanding these hormonal influences can help you tailor your weight loss strategy to your body's needs and cycles.

Psychological Factors

The mental aspect of weight loss is just as important as the physical. Women often face unique psychological challenges related to body image, self-esteem, and societal expectations. Addressing these issues is crucial for long-term success.

- **Body Image**: Society often places immense pressure on women to conform to certain body standards, which can lead to unrealistic expectations and negative self-perception. Cultivating a healthy body image is essential for maintaining motivation and self-compassion throughout your weight loss journey.
- **Emotional Eating**: Women are more likely than men to use food as a coping mechanism for stress, sadness, or boredom. Identifying emotional triggers and finding alternative ways to manage emotions can significantly impact your ability to maintain a healthy diet.
- **Support Systems**: Having a strong support system, whether it's friends, family, or a community of like-minded individuals, can provide encouragement and accountability. Surrounding yourself with positive influences can help you stay motivated and focused on your goals.

Tailoring Your Approach

Recognizing that every woman's body is unique is fundamental to developing an effective weight loss plan. Here are some strategies to consider:

- **Personalized Nutrition**: Work with a nutritionist or dietitian to create a meal plan that meets your individual needs, preferences, and lifestyle. Focus on whole, nutrient-dense foods that provide the energy and nutrients your body needs.
- **Exercise Routine**: Incorporate a mix of cardiovascular exercise, strength training, and flexibility workouts. Find activities that you enjoy and can stick with in the long term.
- **Stress Management**: Practice stress-reducing techniques such as yoga, meditation, or deep breathing exercises. Reducing stress can help regulate cortisol levels and prevent emotional eating.
- **Cycle Syncing**: For women who menstruate, consider aligning your diet and exercise routines with the different phases of your menstrual cycle to optimize energy levels and hormonal balance.

Understanding the unique factors that influence weight loss for women is the foundation of a successful journey. By recognizing the roles of biology, hormones, and psychology, you can create a personalized and sustainable plan that works for you. Remember, weight loss is not a one-size-fits-all process, and the key to success is finding what suits your body, lifestyle, and goals. In the next chapters, we will delve deeper into specific strategies and techniques to help you achieve your health and fitness objectives.

1.1 The Science of Weight Loss

Understanding the science behind weight loss is crucial for making informed decisions about your health and fitness journey. This section will break down the fundamental principles of weight loss, including calorie balance, metabolism, and the roles of macronutrients and micronutrients. Armed with this knowledge, you can develop a strategy that is both effective and sustainable.

Calorie Balance

At its core, weight loss is about creating a calorie deficit, which means consuming fewer calories than your body expends. This concept is often summarized by the simple equation:

Calories In < Calories Out = Weight Loss

- **Calories In**: This represents all the calories you consume through food and beverages. Keeping track of your calorie intake can help you ensure you are not overeating.
- **Calories Out**: This encompasses all the calories your body uses for various functions, including:
  - **Basal Metabolic Rate (BMR)**: The number of calories your body needs at rest to maintain basic physiological functions like breathing, heartbeat, and cell production.
  - **Thermic Effect of Food (TEF)**: The energy required to digest, absorb, and metabolize food. Protein has a higher TEF compared to fats and carbohydrates.
  - **Physical Activity**: Any movement, from structured exercise to daily activities like walking or cleaning.
  - **Non-Exercise Activity Thermogenesis (NEAT)**: Calories burned through non-exercise activities such as fidgeting, standing, or other spontaneous movements.

Creating a calorie deficit can be achieved by reducing calorie intake, increasing physical activity, or a combination of both.

Metabolism

Metabolism is the process through which your body converts the food you eat into energy. It includes all the biochemical reactions that sustain life. Your metabolic rate, or the speed at which these reactions occur, is influenced by several factors:

- **Age**: Metabolic rate typically slows with age, making it easier to gain weight as you get older.
- **Muscle Mass**: Muscle tissue burns more calories than fat tissue, even at rest. Therefore, increasing muscle mass can boost your metabolism.
- **Genetics**: Your genetic makeup plays a role in your metabolic rate, influencing how efficiently your body uses energy.
- **Hormonal Balance**: Hormones such as thyroid hormones, insulin, and cortisol significantly impact metabolism and weight management.

Macronutrients and Micronutrients

Your diet is composed of macronutrients (proteins, carbohydrates, and fats) and micronutrients (vitamins and minerals), each playing a vital role in your overall health and weight loss.

- **Proteins**: Essential for building and repairing tissues, proteins are also crucial for maintaining muscle mass during weight loss. They help you feel full longer, reducing overall calorie intake.
- **Carbohydrates**: The body's primary energy source, carbohydrates should be chosen wisely. Focus on complex carbs like whole grains, vegetables, and legumes, which provide sustained energy and are rich in fiber.
- **Fats**: Healthy fats are necessary for hormone production, nutrient absorption, and cell function. Incorporate sources of unsaturated fats such as avocados, nuts, seeds, and olive oil while limiting saturated and trans fats.
- **Micronutrients**: Vitamins and minerals support a range of bodily functions, from immune response to bone health. A varied diet rich in fruits, vegetables, whole grains, and lean proteins ensures you get the necessary micronutrients.

Energy Expenditure

Understanding how your body expends energy can help you tailor your activities to enhance weight loss. Energy expenditure consists of:

- **Resting Energy Expenditure (REE)**: The calories burned while at rest, account for the majority of your daily energy expenditure.
- **Activity Energy Expenditure (AEE)**: Calories burned through physical activities, including both structured exercise and daily movements.
- **Thermic Effect of Activity (TEA)**: Energy expended during physical exercise. High-intensity workouts burn more calories during and after the activity due to the afterburn effect.

- **Adaptive Thermogenesis**: The body's ability to adapt to different levels of caloric intake and physical activity, which can sometimes slow down weight loss.

The Role of Hormones

Hormones significantly impact weight loss by regulating appetite, metabolism, and fat storage. Key hormones involved in weight management include:

- **Leptin**: Known as the "satiety hormone," leptin helps regulate energy balance by inhibiting hunger. Higher levels of body fat increase leptin levels, but resistance to its effects can lead to overeating.
- **Ghrelin**: Often referred to as the "hunger hormone," ghrelin stimulates appetite. Levels increase before meals and decrease after eating.
- **Insulin**: This hormone regulates blood sugar levels and fat storage. Maintaining stable insulin levels through balanced meals can prevent excessive fat storage and promote weight loss.
- **Cortisol**: Elevated during stress, cortisol can lead to increased appetite and fat storage, particularly around the abdomen. Managing stress through relaxation techniques and adequate sleep can help regulate cortisol levels.

Grasping the science of weight loss equips you with the knowledge to make strategic choices about your diet and lifestyle. Remember that weight loss is a complex interplay of calories, metabolism, nutrients, and hormones. By understanding these components, you can create a personalized plan that addresses your unique needs and challenges, setting the stage for successful and sustainable weight loss. In the next section, we will delve into practical nutrition strategies to help you achieve your health and fitness goals.

1.2 Differences in Male and Female Metabolism

Metabolism is a complex process influenced by numerous factors, including age, muscle mass, hormonal balance, and genetics. While both men and women rely on the same fundamental metabolic processes, there are significant differences in how these processes operate between the sexes. Understanding these differences can help tailor weight loss strategies that are more effective and sustainable for women.

Basal Metabolic Rate (BMR)

Basal Metabolic Rate (BMR) is the number of calories your body needs to maintain basic physiological functions at rest, such as breathing, circulation, and cell production. Several factors contribute to BMR differences between men and women:

- **Muscle Mass**: Men typically have a higher percentage of muscle mass compared to women. Muscle tissue burns more calories than fat tissue, even at rest, resulting in a higher BMR for men. This means men generally require more calories to maintain their body weight.
- **Body Composition**: Women naturally have a higher percentage of body fat compared to men. While fat is essential for reproductive

health and other bodily functions, it does not burn as many calories as muscle. This contributes to a lower BMR in women.

- **Hormonal Differences**: Hormones such as estrogen and progesterone play crucial roles in regulating metabolism and energy expenditure in women. These hormones can affect how efficiently the body burns calories and stores fat.

Hormonal Influences

Hormones significantly impact metabolism and weight management, with distinct differences between men and women:

- **Estrogen and Progesterone**: These hormones fluctuate throughout the menstrual cycle and life stages such as pregnancy and menopause. Estrogen helps regulate fat distribution, often leading to fat storage in the hips and thighs. During menopause, declining estrogen levels can result in increased abdominal fat and a slower metabolism.
- **Testosterone**: Men produce higher levels of testosterone, which supports muscle mass and a higher metabolic rate. Women also produce testosterone, but in smaller amounts, contributing to differences in muscle growth and maintenance.
- **Insulin Sensitivity**: Women and men can differ in their insulin sensitivity, which affects how the body processes and stores glucose. Women with conditions like polycystic ovary syndrome (PCOS) may experience insulin resistance, making weight loss more challenging.
- **Thyroid Hormones**: The thyroid gland regulates metabolism through hormones like thyroxine (T4) and triiodothyronine (T3). Women are more prone to thyroid disorders, such as

hypothyroidism, which can slow metabolism and contribute to weight gain.

Fat Storage and Distribution

The way fat is stored and distributed in the body differs between men and women due to hormonal influences and genetic factors:

- **Women**: Tend to store fat in a gynoid pattern, which means fat accumulates around the hips, thighs, and buttocks. This distribution is partly due to the effects of estrogen. While this pattern is less associated with health risks, it can be more stubborn to lose.
- **Men**: Typically store fat in an android pattern, with fat accumulating around the abdomen. This visceral fat is more metabolically active and linked to higher risks of cardiovascular disease and type 2 diabetes. However, it is often more responsive to diet and exercise interventions.

Energy Expenditure

Daily energy expenditure is influenced by various factors, including physical activity, which can differ between men and women:

- **Activity Levels**: Men often engage in higher-intensity physical activities and have higher overall activity levels, contributing to greater calorie burn. Encouraging women to participate in regular

physical activity, including strength training and high-intensity workouts, can help increase energy expenditure.
- **Non-Exercise Activity Thermogenesis (NEAT)**: NEAT includes all the calories burned through non-exercise activities such as walking, fidgeting, and daily tasks. Women may have lower NEAT due to lifestyle differences, but increasing daily movement can significantly boost calorie expenditure.

Psychological and Behavioral Factors

Behavioral and psychological factors also play a role in how metabolism and weight loss efforts differ between men and women:

- **Dietary Preferences**: Women often prefer different foods and may have unique eating habits compared to men. Understanding these preferences can help in designing personalized nutrition plans that are both enjoyable and effective for weight loss.
- **Stress and Emotional Eating**: Women are more likely to engage in emotional eating, using food as a coping mechanism for stress, sadness, or boredom. This behavior can hinder weight loss efforts and affect metabolic rate. Addressing emotional triggers and finding healthier coping strategies are essential for sustainable weight management.
- **Dieting History**: Women are more likely to have a history of yo-yo dieting, which can affect metabolism. Repeated cycles of weight loss and gain can lead to a slower metabolic rate and make future weight loss more challenging. Emphasizing a balanced, long-term approach to weight management is crucial.

Adaptive Thermogenesis

Adaptive thermogenesis is the body's ability to adjust its energy expenditure in response to changes in diet and physical activity. This adaptive mechanism can be more pronounced in women, making it harder to lose weight:

- **Caloric Restriction**: When women significantly reduce their calorie intake, their bodies may respond by lowering their metabolic rate to conserve energy. This is a survival mechanism but can make weight loss efforts less effective over time.
- **Weight Plateaus**: Women may experience more frequent and prolonged weight loss plateaus due to adaptive thermogenesis. Understanding this natural response can help maintain motivation and adjust strategies as needed.

Strategies to Optimize Female Metabolism

Given the unique aspects of female metabolism, several strategies can help optimize weight loss and overall health:

- **Strength Training**: Incorporating regular strength training exercises helps build muscle mass, which can increase BMR and overall calorie burn. Focus on compound movements that work multiple muscle groups for maximum effectiveness.
- **Balanced Nutrition**: Prioritize a diet rich in whole foods, lean proteins, healthy fats, and complex carbohydrates. Ensure adequate

intake of vitamins and minerals to support overall health and metabolic function.

- **Cycle Syncing**: Align diet and exercise routines with the different phases of the menstrual cycle to optimize energy levels, hormonal balance, and metabolic efficiency.
- **Stress Management**: Practice stress-reducing techniques such as yoga, meditation, and deep breathing exercises. Managing stress can help regulate cortisol levels and prevent emotional eating.
- **Adequate Sleep**: Ensure you get 7-9 hours of quality sleep each night. Sleep plays a critical role in regulating hormones that influence appetite and metabolism, such as leptin and ghrelin.
- **Consistent Physical Activity**: Engage in regular physical activity, including a mix of cardiovascular exercise, strength training, and flexibility workouts. Find activities you enjoy to maintain consistency.
- **Mindful Eating**: Pay attention to hunger and fullness cues, and practice mindful eating to prevent overeating. This can help develop a healthier relationship with food and improve overall dietary habits.

Understanding the differences in male and female metabolism is essential for developing effective and personalized weight loss strategies for women. By considering factors such as hormonal influences, body composition, and psychological aspects, you can create a tailored approach that addresses the unique challenges and opportunities women face in their weight loss journeys. In the next section, we will explore practical nutrition strategies that support female metabolism and promote sustainable weight loss.

1.3 Common Myths and Misconceptions

When it comes to weight loss, misinformation and myths abound, particularly regarding women's health and fitness. These misconceptions can lead to ineffective or even harmful practices. This section aims to debunk some of the most common myths about weight loss for women, providing clarity and evidence-based insights to help you on your journey.

Myth 1: Eating Less Always Leads to Weight Loss

- **The Reality**: While creating a calorie deficit is necessary for weight loss, drastically reducing calorie intake can be counterproductive. Severe calorie restriction can slow down your metabolism as your body shifts into "survival mode," conserving energy and making it harder to lose weight. Additionally, it can lead to nutrient deficiencies, muscle loss, and other health issues.
- **The Better Approach**: Focus on a balanced diet that provides adequate nutrition while maintaining a moderate calorie deficit. Aim for gradual weight loss of 1-2 pounds per week, which is more sustainable and healthier in the long run.

Myth 2: Carbs Are the Enemy

- **The Reality**: Carbohydrates are often vilified in popular diets, but they are a crucial source of energy for your body. The type of carbs you consume matters more than the quantity. Refined carbs and sugars can lead to weight gain and health issues, while complex carbs such as whole grains, fruits, and vegetables provide essential nutrients and fiber.

- **The Better Approach**: Incorporate healthy, complex carbohydrates into your diet. Balance your intake with proteins and fats to maintain steady blood sugar levels and keep you feeling full and energized.

Myth 3: Women Should Avoid Lifting Weights

- **The Reality**: Many women fear that lifting weights will make them bulky or overly muscular. However, women generally do not produce enough testosterone to develop large muscles like men. Strength training is essential for building lean muscle mass, boosting metabolism, and improving overall body composition.
- **The Better Approach**: Include strength training exercises in your fitness routine. Focus on compound movements such as squats, deadlifts, and bench presses, which work multiple muscle groups and provide the most benefit.

Myth 4: Spot Reduction Is Possible

- **The Reality**: Spot reduction, the idea that you can lose fat from specific areas of your body by targeting them with exercises, is a persistent myth. Fat loss occurs throughout the body as you create a calorie deficit, and genetics largely determine where you lose fat first.
- **The Better Approach**: Engage in a balanced exercise regimen that includes both cardiovascular and strength training exercises. This

will help you reduce overall body fat and improve muscle tone in all areas.

Myth 5: Cardio Is the Best Way to Lose Weight

- **The Reality**: While cardiovascular exercise is important for heart health and can help burn calories, relying solely on cardio for weight loss can be less effective than combining it with strength training. Muscle mass increases your resting metabolic rate, helping you burn more calories even when you're not exercising.
- **The Better Approach**: Combine cardio with strength training for a balanced workout routine. Aim for at least 150 minutes of moderate-intensity cardio and two days of strength training per week.

Myth 6: You Have to Eat "Clean" 100% of the Time

- **The Reality**: The notion that you must eat perfectly to lose weight is unrealistic and can lead to feelings of guilt and failure. It's important to maintain a balanced and nutritious diet, but occasional indulgences are part of a healthy lifestyle and can help you maintain your sanity and motivation.
- **The Better Approach**: Follow an 80/20 rule, where 80% of your diet consists of whole, nutrient-dense foods and 20% allows for flexibility and enjoyment. This approach promotes balance and sustainability, reducing the risk of binge eating and other unhealthy behaviors.

Myth 7: Fasted Workouts Burn More Fat

- **The Reality**: While some studies suggest that working out on an empty stomach can increase fat oxidation, it doesn't necessarily translate to greater fat loss over time. Exercising without proper fuel can also lead to decreased performance and muscle loss.
- **The Better Approach**: Listen to your body and eat a small, balanced meal or snack before working out to ensure you have enough energy for a productive session. Post-workout nutrition is also important to aid in recovery and muscle repair.

Myth 8: Supplements Are Necessary for Weight Loss

- **The Reality**: The weight loss supplement industry is vast and often makes exaggerated claims about quick results. Most supplements are not necessary for weight loss and can be ineffective or even harmful if not used correctly.
- **The Better Approach**: Focus on getting your nutrients from a balanced diet. Supplements should only be used to fill in gaps where needed and under the guidance of a healthcare professional. Essential supplements for women might include vitamin D, calcium, and omega-3 fatty acids, but these should complement a healthy diet, not replace it.

Myth 9: You Must Follow a Strict Diet Plan

- **The Reality**: Strict diet plans can be difficult to follow long-term and often lead to feelings of deprivation and eventual relapse.

Flexibility and personalization are key to maintaining a healthy eating pattern.

- **The Better Approach**: Develop a flexible eating plan that suits your lifestyle, preferences, and nutritional needs. Focus on whole foods and listen to your body's hunger and satiety signals. Allow yourself occasional treats to avoid feeling deprived.

Myth 10: Weight Loss Is a Linear Process

- **The Reality**: Weight loss is rarely a straightforward journey. It's normal to experience fluctuations and plateaus along the way. Many factors, including water retention, muscle gain, and hormonal changes, can affect the number on the scale.
- **The Better Approach**: Focus on overall trends rather than daily fluctuations. Use multiple indicators of progress, such as measurements, how your clothes fit, and improvements in fitness levels. Stay patient and consistent with your healthy habits.

Debunking these common myths and misconceptions is crucial for creating a realistic and effective weight loss strategy. By understanding the truths behind these myths, you can make informed decisions that support your health and fitness goals. Remember, weight loss is a personal journey that requires patience, persistence, and self-compassion. In the next section, we will explore practical strategies and techniques to help you achieve your weight loss goals while maintaining a healthy and balanced lifestyle.

1.4 The Importance of Setting Realistic Goals

Setting realistic goals is a cornerstone of successful weight loss. Unrealistic expectations can lead to frustration, disappointment, and ultimately, the abandonment of your weight loss journey. Conversely, attainable goals provide direction, motivation, and a clear path to follow, enhancing your chances of long-term success. This section will guide you through the process of setting realistic goals and explain why they are crucial for achieving and maintaining your health and fitness objectives.

Why Realistic Goals Matter

- **Sustainability**: Unrealistic goals often lead to extreme measures such as crash diets or overly intense exercise routines, which are difficult to maintain and can be harmful to your health. Realistic goals promote gradual, sustainable changes that are more likely to become permanent habits.
- **Motivation and Morale**: Achieving small, realistic goals provides a sense of accomplishment and boosts your confidence. This positive reinforcement keeps you motivated to continue your journey. In contrast, failing to meet unrealistic goals can diminish your morale and lead to discouragement.
- **Health and Well-being**: Rapid weight loss can result in muscle loss, nutritional deficiencies, and other health issues. Realistic goals encourage steady progress that supports overall well-being, allowing your body to adapt and maintain balance.
- **Long-term Success**: Weight loss is not just about shedding pounds quickly; it's about developing a healthier lifestyle. Realistic goals

help you build sustainable habits that contribute to long-term weight management and improved health.

How to Set Realistic Goals

- **Be Specific**: Vague goals like "lose weight" are less effective than specific ones such as "lose 10 pounds in three months." Specific goals provide a clear target and make it easier to track progress.
- **Make Them Measurable**: Ensure your goals are measurable so you can objectively assess your progress. Instead of aiming to "get fitter," set a goal like "run a 5K in under 30 minutes."
- **Achievable**: Set goals that are challenging yet attainable. Consider your current lifestyle, commitments, and resources. For example, if you have a busy schedule, aiming to exercise for 30 minutes three times a week may be more realistic than aiming for daily hour-long sessions.
- **Relevant**: Your goals should align with your overall health and fitness objectives. If your primary aim is to improve cardiovascular health, focus on goals related to aerobic exercise rather than weightlifting.
- **Time-bound**: Give yourself a reasonable timeframe to achieve your goals. This creates a sense of urgency and helps you stay focused. Break down long-term goals into shorter milestones to track your progress and make adjustments as needed.

Examples of Realistic Goals

- **Weight Loss**: Aim to lose 1-2 pounds per week. This rate is generally considered safe and sustainable.

- **Physical Activity**: Start with achievable targets like walking for 30 minutes, five times a week, and gradually increase the duration and intensity.
- **Dietary Changes**: Incorporate one additional serving of vegetables into your daily meals or aim to drink eight glasses of water a day.
- **Fitness Milestones**: Train to complete a specific fitness challenge, such as running a 5K or mastering a particular yoga pose, within a set timeframe.

Tracking and Adjusting Goals

- **Track Your Progress**: Regularly monitor your progress using a journal, app, or other tracking methods. This helps you stay accountable and identify patterns or obstacles.
- **Be Flexible**: Life can be unpredictable, and setbacks are normal. Adjust your goals as needed to accommodate changes in your circumstances. Flexibility ensures you stay on track without becoming discouraged.
- **Celebrate Milestones**: Acknowledge and celebrate your achievements, no matter how small. Recognizing your progress boosts motivation and reinforces positive behavior.

Overcoming Obstacles

- **Identify Barriers**: Reflect on potential challenges that might hinder your progress, such as time constraints, lack of motivation, or emotional eating. Developing strategies to address these barriers in advance can help you stay on course.

- **Seek Support**: Surround yourself with supportive friends, family, or a community of like-minded individuals. Having a support system can provide encouragement, accountability, and practical advice.
- **Stay Positive**: Maintaining a positive mindset is crucial. Focus on what you've achieved rather than what you haven't. Use setbacks as learning opportunities to refine your approach.

Setting realistic goals is essential for a successful weight loss journey. They provide a clear roadmap, keep you motivated, and ensure that your efforts are sustainable and healthy. By being specific, measurable, achievable, relevant, and time-bound in your goal-setting, you can create a solid foundation for lasting change. Remember, the journey to a healthier you is a marathon, not a sprint. In the next section, we will delve into the practical nutrition strategies that will support you in achieving these realistic goals.

Chapter 2: Nutrition Essentials

Nutrition plays a pivotal role in weight loss and overall health. Understanding the basics of nutrition empowers you to make informed choices that fuel your body, support your fitness goals, and enhance your well-being. This chapter will cover essential concepts such as macronutrients, micronutrients, meal planning, and the importance of a balanced diet.

1. Macronutrients: The Building Blocks of Nutrition

Macronutrients are nutrients that your body needs in large amounts to function properly. They provide the energy necessary for daily activities and bodily functions. The three main macronutrients are carbohydrates, proteins, and fats.

Carbohydrates

Carbohydrates are the body's primary source of energy. They are broken down into glucose, which fuels your brain, muscles, and other tissues.

Types of Carbohydrates:

- **Simple Carbohydrates**: Found in sugars, they provide quick energy but can cause rapid spikes and crashes in blood sugar levels.

- **Complex Carbohydrates**: Found in whole grains, vegetables, and legumes, they are digested more slowly, providing sustained energy and stabilizing blood sugar levels.

Healthy Sources:

- Whole grains (brown rice, oats, quinoa)
- Vegetables (broccoli, spinach, sweet potatoes)
- Fruits (apples, berries, bananas)
- Legumes (beans, lentils, chickpeas)

Proteins

Proteins are essential for building and repairing tissues, producing enzymes and hormones, and supporting immune function. They also play a crucial role in preserving muscle mass during weight loss.

Types of Proteins:

Complete Proteins: Contains all nine essential amino acids. Found in animal products and some plant sources like quinoa and soy.

Incomplete Proteins: Lack of one or more essential amino acids. Found in most plant sources.

Healthy Sources:

- Lean meats (chicken, turkey, lean beef)
- Fish and seafood
- Eggs and dairy products
- Plant-based sources (tofu, tempeh, beans, lentils, nuts, seeds)

Fats

Fats are vital for energy, hormone production, nutrient absorption, and protecting organs. They are more calorie-dense than carbohydrates and proteins, so portion control is important.

Types of Fats:

- **Saturated Fats**: Found in animal products and some plant oils. Consume in moderation.
- **Unsaturated Fats**: Include monounsaturated and polyunsaturated fats, found in olive oil, avocados, nuts, and fish. These fats are beneficial for heart health.
- **Trans Fats**: Found in some processed and fried foods. Avoid as much as possible due to their negative health effects.

Healthy Sources:

- Avocados

- Nuts and seeds
- Olive oil and other healthy oils
- Fatty fish (salmon, mackerel, sardines)

2. Micronutrients: Vital Vitamins and Minerals

Micronutrients, including vitamins and minerals, are required in smaller amounts but are crucial for various bodily functions, including immune response, bone health, and energy production.

Essential Vitamins

- **Vitamin A**: Supports vision, immune function, and skin health. Found in carrots, sweet potatoes, and leafy greens.
- **Vitamin C**: Important for immune function, skin health, and antioxidant protection. Found in citrus fruits, strawberries, and bell peppers.
- **Vitamin D**: Crucial for bone health and immune function. Found in fatty fish, fortified dairy products, and through sun exposure.
- **Vitamin E**: Acts as an antioxidant and supports skin and eye health. Found in nuts, seeds, and spinach.
- **Vitamin K**: Important for blood clotting and bone health. Found in leafy greens, broccoli, and Brussels sprouts.

Essential Minerals

- **Calcium**: Necessary for bone health, muscle function, and nerve signaling. Found in dairy products, leafy greens, and fortified plant milks.
- **Iron**: Essential for oxygen transport and energy production. Found in red meat, beans, lentils, and spinach.
- **Magnesium**: Involved in muscle and nerve function, blood sugar control, and bone health. Found in nuts, seeds, and whole grains.
- **Potassium**: Important for heart health, muscle function, and fluid balance. Found in bananas, potatoes, and oranges.
- **Zinc**: Supports immune function, wound healing, and DNA synthesis. Found in meat, shellfish, legumes, and seeds.

3. The Importance of a Balanced Diet

A balanced diet provides the right proportions of macronutrients and micronutrients to support your body's needs. It ensures you get enough energy for daily activities and enough nutrients to maintain overall health.

Components of a Balanced Diet:

- **Variety**: Eating a wide range of foods ensures you get a diverse array of nutrients.
- **Moderation**: Control portion sizes to avoid overeating and ensure calorie intake aligns with your goals.

- **Proportionality**: Balance different food groups to meet your nutritional needs. Follow guidelines such as the MyPlate model, which emphasizes fruits, vegetables, grains, protein, and dairy.

4. Meal Planning and Preparation

Effective meal planning and preparation can help you stay on track with your nutritional goals, save time, and reduce the temptation to make unhealthy food choices.

Steps for Successful Meal Planning

- **Set Goals**: Determine your nutritional needs and weight loss goals. Plan meals that align with these objectives.
- **Create a Schedule**: Decide how many meals and snacks you need each day. Plan your menu for the week to ensure variety and balance.
- **Make a Shopping List**: Write down the ingredients you need for your planned meals. Stick to the list to avoid impulse purchases.
- **Prep in Advance**: Prepare ingredients or entire meals ahead of time. This can include chopping vegetables, cooking grains, and portioning out snacks.
- **Stay Flexible**: Be prepared to adjust your meal plan based on the availability of ingredients, time constraints, and changing preferences.

5. Hydration and Its Role in Weight Loss

Staying hydrated is crucial for overall health and can support weight loss efforts. Water is involved in digestion, nutrient absorption, and waste elimination.

Benefits of Proper Hydration:

- **Appetite Control**: Drinking water before meals can help you feel full and reduce calorie intake.
- **Metabolism Boost**: Adequate hydration supports metabolic processes, helping your body burn calories more efficiently.
- **Energy Levels**: Staying hydrated can prevent fatigue and improve physical performance, making it easier to stay active.

Tips for Staying Hydrated:

- Drink a glass of water upon waking and before each meal.
- Carry a reusable water bottle to remind yourself to drink throughout the day.
- Incorporate water-rich foods such as fruits and vegetables into your diet.

Understanding nutrition essentials is the foundation of any successful weight loss journey. By focusing on the right balance of macronutrients and micronutrients, planning and preparing your meals, and staying hydrated, you can support your body's needs and achieve your health and fitness goals. In the next chapter, we will explore effective exercise strategies to complement your nutrition plan and maximize your weight loss efforts.

2.1 Balanced Diet Fundamentals

A balanced diet is the cornerstone of good health and effective weight loss. It ensures your body receives the essential nutrients it needs to function optimally while supporting your fitness goals. This section will delve into the fundamentals of a balanced diet, focusing on how to create meals that provide the right proportions of macronutrients and micronutrients.

What is a Balanced Diet?

A balanced diet includes a variety of foods in the right proportions to provide your body with the necessary nutrients for energy, growth, and maintenance of bodily functions. It encompasses the following key components:

- **Carbohydrates**: Should make up about 45-65% of your total daily calories. Focus on complex carbohydrates like whole grains, fruits, and vegetables.
- **Proteins**: Should account for 10-35% of your daily calories. Include a mix of animal and plant-based protein sources.
- **Fats**: Should comprise 20-35% of your daily calories. Prioritize healthy fats from sources like avocados, nuts, seeds, and fish.

- **Vitamins and Minerals**: Ensure you consume a variety of foods to meet your micronutrient needs, including vitamins A, C, D, E, K, and B-complex, along with minerals like calcium, iron, magnesium, and potassium.
- **Fiber**: Aim for at least 25-30 grams of fiber per day from fruits, vegetables, whole grains, and legumes.
- **Water**: Stay hydrated by drinking plenty of water throughout the day.

Building a Balanced Plate

The key to a balanced diet is creating meals that include a variety of foods from different food groups. The MyPlate model, developed by the USDA, is a helpful guide for building a balanced plate:

- **Half Your Plate Fruits and Vegetables**: Aim for a variety of colors and types to ensure you get a wide range of nutrients. Vegetables should make up the larger portion.
- **One Quarter Whole Grains**: Choose whole grains like brown rice, quinoa, oats, and whole wheat bread. These provide essential fiber and nutrients.
- **One-Quarter Protein**: Include lean protein sources such as chicken, fish, beans, lentils, tofu, and low-fat dairy.
- **Include Healthy Fats**: Add small amounts of healthy fats to your meals, such as olive oil, nuts, seeds, and avocados.

Portion Control

Portion control is vital for managing calorie intake and preventing overeating. Even healthy foods can contribute to weight gain if consumed in excessive amounts. Here are some tips for portion control:

- **Use Smaller Plates**: This can help you feel satisfied with smaller portions.
- **Read Labels**: Pay attention to serving sizes on food labels and measure portions accordingly.
- **Listen to Your Body**: Eat slowly and pay attention to hunger and fullness cues. Stop eating when you feel satisfied, not stuffed.
- **Pre-portion Snacks**: Divide snacks into single-serving portions to avoid mindless eating.

Meal Timing and Frequency

How often and when you eat can also affect your metabolism and energy levels. While there's no one-size-fits-all approach, consider these general guidelines:

- **Regular Meals**: Eating regular meals throughout the day can help maintain energy levels and prevent overeating. Aim for three balanced meals and one or two healthy snacks if needed.
- **Breakfast**: A nutritious breakfast can kickstart your metabolism and provide energy for the day. Include a mix of protein, complex carbohydrates, and healthy fats.

- **Evening Meals**: Avoid heavy, calorie-dense meals late at night. Opt for lighter, nutrient-dense options in the evening.

The Role of Variety in a Balanced Diet

Variety is crucial for ensuring you get a broad spectrum of nutrients. Eating a wide range of foods also keeps your meals interesting and enjoyable. Here are some tips to add variety:

- **Rotate Foods**: Regularly switch up your protein sources, grains, and vegetables.
- **Try New Recipes**: Experiment with new recipes and cooking methods to keep your diet exciting.
- **Seasonal Produce**: Incorporate seasonal fruits and vegetables into your meals for freshness and variety.

Mindful Eating

Mindful eating involves paying attention to what you eat and savoring each bite. This practice can help you make healthier choices and enjoy your food more:

- **Eat Without Distractions**: Avoid eating while watching TV or using electronic devices.
- **Chew Thoroughly**: Take time to chew your food well, which aids digestion and helps you feel full.

- **Appreciate Your Food**: Take a moment to appreciate the flavors, textures, and smells of your meal.

A balanced diet is fundamental to achieving your weight loss and health goals. By focusing on the right mix of macronutrients and micronutrients, practicing portion control, and incorporating variety and mindful eating into your routine, you can support your body's needs and enjoy a healthier lifestyle. In the next section, we will explore practical meal planning and preparation tips to help you implement these principles effectively.

2.2 Macronutrients: Proteins, Carbs, and Fats

Macronutrients are the main nutrients your body needs in large amounts to function properly. They provide energy (calories) and are essential for growth, metabolism, and overall health. Understanding the roles and sources of proteins, carbohydrates, and fats can help you create a balanced diet that supports your weight loss and fitness goals.

Proteins

Proteins are crucial for building and repairing tissues, producing enzymes and hormones, and supporting immune function. They are made up of amino acids, often referred to as the building blocks of proteins.

Sources of Protein:

- **Animal Sources**: Include lean meats (chicken, turkey, lean cuts of beef and pork), fish, eggs, and dairy products (milk, yogurt, cheese).
- **Plant Sources**: Legumes (beans, lentils, chickpeas), tofu, tempeh, edamame, quinoa, nuts, seeds, and some whole grains (such as quinoa and farro).

Role in Weight Loss: Protein is important for preserving lean muscle mass while losing weight. It also helps you feel full and satisfied after meals, which can prevent overeating.

Recommended Intake: The recommended dietary allowance (RDA) for protein is about 0.8 grams per kilogram of body weight, but this can vary based on individual needs, activity level, and goals.

Carbohydrates

Carbohydrates are the body's primary source of energy. They are broken down into glucose (blood sugar), which fuels your brain, muscles, and other tissues. There are two main types of carbohydrates:

1. Complex Carbohydrates:

- Found in whole grains (brown rice, oats, quinoa), vegetables (sweet potatoes, leafy greens), and legumes (beans, lentils).

- Provide sustained energy and contains fiber, which supports digestive health and helps you feel full.

2. Simple Carbohydrates:

- Found in sugars (table sugar, honey, syrups) and refined grains (white bread, white rice).
- Provides quick energy but can cause rapid spikes and crashes in blood sugar levels.

Role in Weight Loss: Choosing complex carbohydrates over simple carbohydrates can help stabilize blood sugar levels and promote feelings of fullness, which may aid in weight management.

Recommended Intake: Carbohydrate needs vary based on factors such as activity level and metabolism. Focus on whole, unprocessed sources and adjust intake based on individual goals.

Fats

Fats are essential for energy, hormone production, nutrient absorption (such as fat-soluble vitamins A, D, E, and K), and protecting organs. There are different types of fats, each with varying effects on health:

1. Unsaturated Fats:

- **Monounsaturated Fats**: Found in olive oil, avocados, nuts (such as almonds, and peanuts), and seeds (such as sunflower seeds).
- **Polyunsaturated Fats**: Found in fatty fish (salmon, trout), flaxseeds, chia seeds, and walnuts.
- These fats are beneficial for heart health and can help lower LDL (bad) cholesterol levels when consumed in place of saturated and trans fats.

2. Saturated Fats:

- Found in animal products (fatty cuts of meat, poultry with skin, whole-fat dairy) and some plant oils (coconut oil, palm oil).
- Consuming too much-saturated fat can increase LDL cholesterol levels and risk of heart disease. Limit intake and choose leaner options when possible.

2. Trans Fats:

- Found in processed foods (such as snack cakes, and fried foods) and some margarines.
- Trans fats are the most harmful type of fat and should be avoided as much as possible due to their negative impact on heart health.

Role in Weight Loss: Including healthy fats in your diet can help you feel satisfied after meals and support overall health. They also provide essential fatty acids that your body cannot produce on its own.

Recommended Intake: Aim to include mostly unsaturated fats in your diet, limiting saturated fats and avoiding trans fats as much as possible. Moderation is key, as fats are calorie-dense.

Proteins, carbohydrates, and fats are essential macronutrients that play distinct roles in your diet and overall health. By choosing a balanced combination of these nutrients from wholesome sources, you can support your weight loss goals while ensuring your body gets the energy and nutrients it needs to thrive. In the next section, we will explore practical tips for meal planning and preparation to help you incorporate these macronutrients into your daily meals effectively.

2.3 Micronutrients: Vitamins and Minerals

Micronutrients are essential nutrients required by the body in small amounts but play critical roles in various physiological functions, including metabolism, immune function, and overall health. Vitamins and minerals are the two main categories of micronutrients, each contributing uniquely to your well-being.

Vitamins

Vitamins are organic compounds that are essential for normal growth and nutrition. They are classified into two main categories based on their solubility:

1. Fat-Soluble Vitamins:

- **Vitamin A**: Supports vision, immune function, and skin health. Found in orange and yellow vegetables (carrots, sweet potatoes), spinach, and liver.
- **Vitamin D**: Crucial for bone health and immune function. Synthesized by the skin when exposed to sunlight and found in fatty fish (salmon, mackerel), egg yolks, and fortified dairy products.
- **Vitamin E**: Acts as an antioxidant, protecting cells from damage. Found in nuts (almonds, hazelnuts), seeds (sunflower seeds, pumpkin seeds), and vegetable oils (sunflower oil, safflower oil).
- **Vitamin K**: Important for blood clotting and bone health. Found in leafy greens (spinach, kale), broccoli, and Brussels sprouts.

2. Water-Soluble Vitamins:

- **Vitamin C**: Supports immune function, wound healing, and antioxidant protection. Found in citrus fruits (oranges, lemons), strawberries, bell peppers, and broccoli.
- **Vitamin B Complex**: Includes several vitamins that play roles in energy metabolism, nervous system function, and red blood cell production.

  - B1 (Thiamine): Found in whole grains, pork, and legumes.
  - B2 (Riboflavin): Found in dairy products, lean meats, and leafy greens.
  - B3 (Niacin): Found in poultry, fish, nuts, and whole grains.
  - B6 (Pyridoxine): Found in potatoes, bananas, and chickpeas.

- B12 (Cobalamin): Found in animal products (meat, fish, dairy) and fortified plant-based foods (nutritional yeast, fortified cereals).

Minerals

Minerals are inorganic elements essential for various bodily functions, including bone health, fluid balance, nerve function, and muscle contraction. They are categorized into two groups based on their required intake:

1. Major Minerals (Macrominerals):

- **Calcium**: Critical for bone health, muscle function, and nerve transmission. Found in dairy products, leafy greens (kale, collard greens), and fortified plant milks.
- **Magnesium**: Supports muscle and nerve function, blood sugar regulation, and bone health. Found in nuts (almonds, cashews), seeds (pumpkin seeds, sunflower seeds), and whole grains.
- **Potassium**: Important for heart health, muscle function, and electrolyte balance. Found in bananas, potatoes, citrus fruits, and leafy greens.
- **Sodium**: Important for fluid balance and nerve function. Found in table salt and processed foods, but excess intake should be limited.

2. Trace Minerals:

- **Iron**: Essential for oxygen transport and energy production. Found in red meat, poultry, fish, legumes (beans, lentils), and fortified cereals.
- **Zinc**: Supports immune function, wound healing, and protein synthesis. Found in oysters, red meat, poultry, and fortified cereals.
- **Selenium**: Acts as an antioxidant and supports thyroid function. Found in Brazil nuts, seafood, and whole grains.
- **Iodine**: Crucial for thyroid function and hormone production. Found in iodized salt, seafood, and dairy products.

Importance of Micronutrients in Weight Loss

Micronutrients play a vital role in supporting metabolism, energy production, and overall health during weight loss. Deficiencies in certain vitamins and minerals can impair metabolic processes and energy levels, making it harder to achieve and maintain a healthy weight.

Tips for Ensuring Micronutrient Adequacy:

- **Eat a Variety of Foods**: Incorporate a diverse range of fruits, vegetables, whole grains, lean proteins, and healthy fats into your diet.
- **Consider Supplements**: If you have specific dietary restrictions or health conditions, consult with a healthcare provider to determine if supplements are necessary.

- **Avoid Highly Processed Foods**: These foods often lack essential nutrients and may contribute to nutrient deficiencies over time.

Micronutrients, including vitamins and minerals, are essential for overall health and well-being. They support numerous bodily functions and play critical roles in metabolism and energy production, which are important for achieving and maintaining a healthy weight. By consuming a balanced diet rich in nutrient-dense foods, you can ensure you meet your micronutrient needs and support your weight loss goals effectively. In the next section, we will explore practical strategies for meal planning and preparation to help you incorporate these vital micronutrients into your daily meals.

2.4 Meal Planning and Preparation

Meal planning and preparation are key strategies for achieving and maintaining a balanced diet that supports your weight loss and health goals. By taking the time to plan your meals and prep ingredients in advance, you can save time, make healthier choices, and ensure you have nutritious meals readily available throughout the week.

Benefits of Meal Planning

1. **Saves Time**: Planning your meals reduces the time spent deciding what to eat and preparing meals each day.
2. **Promotes Healthy Choices**: By planning, you're more likely to choose nutritious ingredients and balanced meals rather than opting for convenient, less healthy options.

3. **Reduces Food Waste**: Planning helps you buy only what you need and use ingredients efficiently, reducing food waste.
4. **Supports Weight Management**: With a meal plan, you can control portion sizes and ensure your meals align with your calorie and nutrient needs.

Steps for Effective Meal Planning

1. **Set Goals and Consider Preferences:**

- Determine your nutritional goals, such as calorie intake, macronutrient distribution (protein, carbs, fats), and dietary preferences (vegetarian, gluten-free).
- Consider your schedule and lifestyle to plan meals that are practical and enjoyable.

2. **Create a Weekly Meal Plan:**

- Plan your meals for the week, including breakfast, lunch, dinner, and snacks. Use a template or calendar to organize your plan.
- Include a variety of foods to ensure you get a diverse range of nutrients. Balance meals with protein, complex carbohydrates, healthy fats, and plenty of fruits and vegetables.

3. **Make a Shopping List:**

- Based on your meal plan, create a shopping list of ingredients you'll need for the week.
- Organize your list by food categories (produce, proteins, pantry items) to streamline your shopping trip.

4. Prep Ingredients:

- Dedicate time to prep ingredients in advance, such as washing and chopping vegetables, cooking grains or proteins, and portioning out snacks.
- Store prepped ingredients in air-tight containers or storage bags for easy access during meal preparation.

5. Cook and Store Meals:

- Cook meals in batches, especially for items that can be easily reheated or assembled quickly during the week.
- Use portion-controlled containers to store meals and snacks in the refrigerator or freezer for later consumption.

Tips for Meal Preparation

1. **Batch Cooking**: Prepare larger batches of meals that can be portioned and stored for multiple meals throughout the week.
2. **Use Kitchen Tools**: Invest in time-saving kitchen tools such as a slow cooker, instant pot, or food processor to streamline meal preparation.

3. **Choose Nutrient-Dense Foods**: Prioritize nutrient-dense foods like lean proteins, whole grains, fruits, and vegetables in your meal plan.
4. **Be Flexible**: Allow for flexibility in your meal plan to accommodate changes in schedule or preferences. Use leftovers creatively to reduce food waste.
5. **Monitor Portion Sizes**: Use portion-control tools such as measuring cups, spoons, and kitchen scales to ensure you're consuming appropriate portion sizes.

Incorporating Micronutrients

1. **Include a Variety of Colors**: Aim for meals that include a variety of colorful fruits and vegetables to ensure you're getting a range of vitamins and minerals.
2. **Choose Whole Foods**: Opt for whole grains, lean proteins, and healthy fats to maximize nutrient intake and support overall health.
3. **Consider Supplements**: If needed, consult with a healthcare provider to determine if supplements are necessary to meet your specific nutrient needs.

Meal planning and preparation are valuable tools for achieving your weight loss and health goals. By taking the time to plan nutritious meals, shop for ingredients, and prep in advance, you can make healthier choices, save time, and support your overall well-being. These practices not only simplify your daily eating habits but also ensure you're meeting your nutritional needs effectively. In the next section, we will explore effective strategies for incorporating physical activity into your lifestyle to complement your nutrition plan and maximize your weight loss efforts.

2.5 Healthy and Delicious Recipes

Eating nutritious meals doesn't have to be bland. Incorporating healthy and delicious recipes into your meal plan can make achieving your weight loss and health goals enjoyable and satisfying. Below are a few recipes that are not only nutritious but also flavorful and easy to prepare:

1. Quinoa and Vegetable Stir-Fry

Ingredients:

- 1 cup quinoa, rinsed
- 2 cups water or vegetable broth
- 1 tablespoon olive oil
- 1 onion, diced
- 2 cloves garlic, minced
- 1 bell pepper, diced (any color)
- 1 zucchini, diced
- 1 cup broccoli florets
- 1 carrot, sliced
- Soy sauce or tamari, to taste
- Salt and pepper, to taste
- Optional: tofu or cooked chicken for added protein

Instructions:

- In a medium saucepan, bring the water or vegetable broth to a boil. Add quinoa, reduce heat to low, cover, and simmer for 15-20 minutes, or until quinoa is cooked and liquid is absorbed.
- In a large skillet or wok, heat olive oil over medium-high heat. Add onion and garlic, and sauté until softened.
- Add bell pepper, zucchini, broccoli, and carrot to the skillet. Cook, stirring frequently, until vegetables are tender-crisp.
- Add cooked quinoa to the skillet with the vegetables. Stir in soy sauce or tamari, salt, and pepper to taste. Cook for an additional 2-3 minutes to heat through.
- Serve hot, optionally topped with tofu or cooked chicken for added protein.

2. Grilled Lemon Herb Chicken with Quinoa Salad

Ingredients:

- 4 boneless, skinless chicken breasts
- Juice of 1 lemon
- 2 tablespoons olive oil
- 2 cloves garlic, minced
- 1 teaspoon dried oregano
- 1 teaspoon dried thyme
- Salt and pepper, to taste

Quinoa Salad:

- 1 cup quinoa, rinsed
- 2 cups water or chicken broth
- 1 cucumber, diced
- 1 tomato, diced
- 1/4 cup red onion, finely chopped
- Handful of fresh parsley, chopped
- Juice of 1 lemon
- 2 tablespoons olive oil
- Salt and pepper, to taste

Instructions:

- In a bowl, combine lemon juice, olive oil, minced garlic, dried oregano, dried thyme, salt, and pepper. Mix well.
- Place chicken breasts in a resealable plastic bag or shallow dish. Pour the marinade over the chicken, coating evenly. Marinate in the refrigerator for at least 30 minutes (or overnight for best flavor).
- Cook quinoa: In a medium saucepan, bring water or chicken broth to a boil. Add quinoa, reduce heat to low, cover, and simmer for 15-20 minutes, or until quinoa is cooked and liquid is absorbed. Fluff with a fork and let cool.
- Preheat the grill or grill pan over medium-high heat. Grill chicken breasts for 6-7 minutes per side, or until internal temperature reaches 165°F (75°C) and juices run clear.
- Prepare quinoa salad: In a large bowl, combine cooked quinoa, diced cucumber, tomato, red onion, and chopped parsley. Dress with lemon juice, olive oil, salt, and pepper. Toss to combine.
- Serve grilled lemon herb chicken alongside quinoa salad. Garnish with additional fresh herbs if desired.

3. Spinach and Feta Stuffed Bell Peppers

Ingredients:

- 4 bell peppers, any color
- 1 tablespoon olive oil
- 1 onion, diced
- 2 cloves garlic, minced
- 5 cups fresh spinach, chopped
- 1 cup cooked quinoa or brown rice
- 1/2 cup crumbled feta cheese
- Salt and pepper, to taste
- Optional: chopped fresh herbs (such as parsley or basil)

Instructions:

- Preheat oven to 375°F (190°C). Grease a baking dish with olive oil or non-stick cooking spray.
- Cut the tops off the bell peppers and remove seeds and membranes. Place peppers upright in the prepared baking dish.
- In a large skillet, heat olive oil over medium heat. Add onion and garlic, and sauté until softened.
- Add chopped spinach to the skillet, and cook until wilted. Stir in cooked quinoa or brown rice, crumbled feta cheese, salt, and pepper. Cook for 2-3 minutes to combine flavors.
- Spoon the spinach and quinoa mixture evenly into the hollowed-out bell peppers.

- Cover the baking dish with foil and bake for 30-35 minutes, or until bell peppers are tender.
- Remove from oven and sprinkle with optional chopped fresh herbs before serving.

Tips for Delicious and Nutritious Meals

- Use Fresh Ingredients: Opt for fresh produce and lean proteins to maximize flavor and nutrition.
- Experiment with Herbs and Spices: Enhance the taste of your dishes with fresh herbs like basil, parsley, or cilantro, and spices such as cumin, paprika, or turmeric.
- Balance Macronutrients: Include a balance of protein, carbohydrates, and healthy fats in each meal to keep you satisfied and energized.
- Portion Control: Pay attention to portion sizes to ensure you're meeting your nutritional goals without overeating.

Enjoy these recipes as part of your balanced diet, and feel free to customize them based on your preferences and dietary needs. Healthy eating can be delicious and rewarding, supporting your journey to achieve and maintain a healthy weight.

Chapter 3: Effective Exercise Strategies

In addition to maintaining a balanced diet, incorporating effective exercise strategies into your routine is crucial for achieving and sustaining weight loss, improving overall fitness, and enhancing your well-being. This chapter explores various exercise principles and strategies tailored specifically for women, focusing on maximizing results and promoting a healthy lifestyle.

1. Benefits of Exercise for Women

Regular physical activity offers numerous benefits beyond weight management. For women, exercise:

- **Promotes Weight Loss**: Helps burn calories and fat, supporting weight loss goals.
- **Improves Cardiovascular Health**: Reduces the risk of heart disease, stroke, and hypertension.
- **Enhances Muscle Tone**: Builds and tones muscles, improving overall strength and endurance.
- **Boosts Mood and Mental Health**: Releases endorphins that reduce stress, anxiety, and symptoms of depression.
- **Supports Bone Health**: Helps maintain bone density and reduces the risk of osteoporosis.
- **Enhances Sleep Quality**: Promotes deeper, more restorative sleep patterns.

2. Types of Exercise for Women

Cardiovascular Exercise:

Benefits: Improves heart health, burns calories, and enhances endurance.

Examples: Walking, jogging, cycling, swimming, aerobics, dancing.

Strength Training:

Benefits: Builds lean muscle mass, boosts metabolism, and enhances strength.

Examples: Weightlifting, resistance band exercises, bodyweight exercises (squats, push-ups).

Flexibility and Stretching:

Benefits: Improves range of motion, reduces muscle stiffness, and prevents injuries.

Examples: Yoga, Pilates, static stretching exercises.

Functional Training:

Benefits: Enhances balance, stability, and coordination for everyday activities.

Examples: Core exercises, balance exercises, functional movements (lunges, planks).

3. Designing an Effective Exercise Program

Set Realistic Goals:

Define specific goals such as weight loss, muscle gain, or improved fitness levels.

Choose Activities You Enjoy:

Incorporate exercises that you find enjoyable and sustainable for long-term adherence.

Create a Balanced Routine:

Include a mix of cardiovascular, strength training, flexibility, and functional exercises.

Gradually Increase Intensity:

Progressively challenge your body by increasing weights, speed, or duration of exercises.

Schedule Regular Exercise Sessions:

Aim for at least 150 minutes of moderate-intensity aerobic activity or 75 minutes of vigorous-intensity activity per week, plus muscle-strengthening activities on two or more days.

4. Tips for Effective Exercise

Warm-Up and Cool Down:

Always start with a warm-up to prepare your muscles and joints, and finish with a cool-down to promote recovery.

Stay Hydrated:

Drink water before, during, and after exercise to stay hydrated and maintain performance.

Use Proper Form and Technique:

Focus on correct form to prevent injuries and maximize effectiveness of exercises.

Listen to Your Body:

Pay attention to how your body feels and adjust exercise intensity or type as needed.

Incorporate Variety:

Keep your routine interesting and prevent plateaus by varying exercises and activities.

5. Overcoming Barriers to Exercise

- **Time Constraints**: Schedule workouts into your daily routine and prioritize physical activity.
- **Lack of Motivation**: Find a workout buddy, join group classes, or set achievable goals to stay motivated.
- **Injury or Health Concerns**: Consult with a healthcare professional for exercise modifications or alternatives.
- **Weather Conditions**: Have indoor exercise options or adapt activities to different seasons.
- **Mental Barriers**: Practice mindfulness techniques, set realistic expectations, and celebrate progress.

Effective exercise strategies are essential for women to achieve their weight loss, fitness, and health goals. By incorporating a balanced exercise program that includes cardiovascular, strength training, flexibility, and functional exercises, you can improve overall well-being and maintain a healthy lifestyle. Consistency, enjoyment, and proper technique are key factors in maximizing the benefits of exercise. In the following chapters, we will delve into specific tips and guidance for overcoming common challenges, staying motivated, and integrating exercise seamlessly into your daily life.

3.1 Cardio Workouts: Benefits and Types

Cardiovascular exercise, often referred to as cardio, plays a pivotal role in improving overall fitness, aiding weight loss efforts, and enhancing cardiovascular health. This section explores the benefits of cardio workouts specifically for women and outlines various types of cardio exercises to incorporate into your fitness regimen.

Benefits of Cardio Workouts for Women

- **Improves Heart Health**: Cardio exercises strengthen the heart muscle, improve circulation, and lower blood pressure, reducing the risk of heart disease.
- **Aids Weight Loss**: Regular cardio helps burn calories and fat, promoting weight loss and weight management when combined with a balanced diet.
- **Enhances Endurance**: Builds stamina and endurance, allowing you to perform daily activities with less fatigue.
- **Boosts Mood**: Releases endorphins, chemicals that reduce stress and anxiety while promoting a sense of well-being and relaxation.
- **Increases Energy Levels**: Improves oxygen flow to muscles and tissues, enhancing overall energy levels and combating feelings of fatigue.

- **Supports Better Sleep**: Promotes deeper and more restful sleep, which is essential for overall health and recovery.

Types of Cardio Exercises

- **Walking**: A low-impact activity that can be done anywhere, from neighborhoods to nature trails. It's suitable for all fitness levels and easy to incorporate into daily routines.
- **Running/Jogging**: Increases cardiovascular endurance and burns calories efficiently. It can be done outdoors or on a treadmill, offering versatility in intensity and terrain.
- **Cycling**: Whether outdoors or on a stationary bike, cycling strengthens the legs and improves cardiovascular fitness while being gentle on the joints.
- **Swimming**: Provides a full-body workout that builds endurance, strength, and flexibility. It's especially beneficial for those with joint issues or injuries.
- **Dancing**: Engages the entire body while making exercise fun and enjoyable. Various dance styles, from Zumba to hip-hop, offer cardio benefits while improving coordination and rhythm.
- **Jump Rope**: A portable and effective cardio workout that enhances coordination and agility while burning a significant amount of calories in a short time.
- **Group Fitness Classes**: Includes options like aerobics, kickboxing, and dance-based workouts. These classes offer motivation, variety, and social interaction while delivering a challenging cardio workout.
- **High-Intensity Interval Training (HIIT)**: Alternates between short bursts of intense activity followed by periods of rest or

lower-intensity exercise. HIIT boosts metabolism, improves cardiovascular fitness, and can be adapted to various fitness levels.

Incorporating Cardio Workouts into Your Routine

- **Frequency**: Aim for at least 150 minutes of moderate-intensity cardio exercise per week, or 75 minutes of vigorous-intensity exercise spread across the week.
- **Intensity**: Adjust the intensity based on your fitness level and goals. Beginners may start with low to moderate intensity and gradually increase as fitness improves.
- **Variety**: Incorporate different types of cardio exercises to prevent boredom, challenge different muscle groups, and avoid overuse injuries.
- **Progression**: Gradually increase the duration, intensity, or frequency of workouts to continue challenging your cardiovascular system and improving fitness levels.

Cardiovascular workouts are essential for women's health and fitness, offering a range of benefits from improved heart health and weight management to enhanced mood and energy levels. By incorporating various types of cardio exercises into your routine and adjusting intensity and duration as needed, you can achieve optimal fitness and overall well-being. In the next section, we will explore effective strategies for incorporating strength training to complement your cardio regimen and achieve comprehensive fitness goals.

3.2 Strength Training for Women

Strength training, also known as resistance training or weight training, involves exercises designed to improve muscular strength, endurance, and tone. This section explores the benefits of strength training specifically for women, dispels common myths, and provides practical guidance on how to incorporate strength training into your fitness routine effectively.

Benefits of Strength Training for Women

- **Increases Muscle Strength**: Strength training builds and strengthens muscles, which is particularly beneficial for women to maintain bone density and reduce the risk of osteoporosis.
- **Boosts Metabolism**: Muscle tissue burns more calories than fat tissue, so increasing muscle mass through strength training can help enhance metabolism and support weight management.
- **Improves Body Composition**: Helps reduce body fat percentage and increase lean muscle mass, leading to a more toned and defined physique.
- **Enhances Functional Strength**: Improves muscular endurance and strength, making daily activities easier and reducing the risk of injury.
- **Promotes Bone Health**: Weight-bearing exercises stimulate bone growth and help maintain bone density, crucial for preventing osteoporosis.
- **Supports Joint Health**: Strengthens muscles around joints, improving stability and reducing the risk of joint injuries and pain.

Common Myths about Strength Training for Women

- **Myth: Strength training will make women bulky.**

Fact: Women typically have lower levels of testosterone compared to men, which is essential for significant muscle hypertrophy (growth). Strength training tones muscles and enhances definition without causing excessive bulkiness.

- **Myth: Strength training is only for young women or athletes.**

Fact: Strength training is beneficial for women of all ages and fitness levels. It helps maintain muscle mass, bone density, and functional strength as you age.

- **Myth: Cardio is more effective than strength training for weight loss.**

Fact: While cardio burns calories during exercise, strength training increases metabolism and burns calories even at rest, supporting long-term weight management and body composition changes.

How to Incorporate Strength Training into Your Routine

1. **Start with a Warm-Up**: Begin each session with a 5-10 minute warm-up to increase blood flow to muscles and prepare your body for exercise.

2. **Choose Your Exercises:**

- **Compound Exercises**: Work multiple muscle groups simultaneously, such as squats, deadlifts, lunges, and push-ups.
- **Isolation Exercises**: Target specific muscles, like bicep curls, tricep extensions, and calf raises.

3. **Progression and Resistance:**

- Gradually increase the weight or resistance as your strength improves to continue challenging your muscles.
- Aim for 2-3 sets of 8-12 repetitions per exercise, adjusting the weight to reach fatigue by the final few repetitions.

4. **Focus on Proper Form:**

- Maintain correct posture and technique throughout each exercise to prevent injury and maximize effectiveness.
- Consider working with a certified personal trainer to learn proper form and technique, especially when starting.

5. Rest and Recovery:

- Allow muscles time to recover between sessions, typically 48 hours for each muscle group.
- Include stretching or yoga to enhance flexibility and reduce muscle soreness.

6. Consistency is Key:

- Aim for 2-3 strength training sessions per week, alternating between different muscle groups to allow adequate recovery.

Incorporating Strength Training with Cardio

- **Balanced Routine**: Combine strength training with cardiovascular exercises to achieve a well-rounded fitness program.
- **Schedule**: Alternate strength training days with cardio or incorporate both types of exercises within the same session, based on your fitness goals and preferences.

By incorporating proper technique, progression, and consistency into your strength training regimen, you can achieve significant fitness gains and support long-term wellness. In the next chapter, we will discuss strategies for integrating flexibility and mobility exercises to enhance your overall fitness and ensure well-rounded physical health.

3.3 Flexibility and Mobility Exercises

Flexibility and mobility exercises are essential components of a well-rounded fitness routine for women, contributing to improved range of motion, reduced risk of injury, and enhanced overall physical performance. This section explores the benefits of flexibility and mobility exercises, provides examples of effective stretches, and offers practical tips for integrating them into your fitness regimen.

Benefits of Flexibility and Mobility Exercises

- **Improved Range of Motion**: Stretching exercises help lengthen muscles and tendons, enhancing flexibility and allowing joints to move through their full range of motion.
- **Reduced Muscle Tension and Stiffness**: Regular stretching reduces muscle tightness and stiffness, promoting relaxation and improving posture.
- **Enhanced Athletic Performance**: Improved flexibility and mobility contribute to better agility, coordination, and athletic performance in various activities.
- **Injury Prevention**: Flexible muscles and joints are less prone to strains, sprains, and other injuries during physical activities and daily tasks.
- **Better Posture and Balance**: Stretching exercises improve muscle balance and alignment, supporting better posture and reducing the risk of falls.
- **Mind-Body Connection**: Stretching promotes relaxation, reduces stress, and enhances mindfulness by focusing on breathing and body awareness.

Types of Flexibility and Mobility Exercises

- **Static Stretching**: Hold each stretch at the point of mild tension for 15-30 seconds, focusing on major muscle groups such as hamstrings, quadriceps, calves, and shoulders.
- **Dynamic Stretching**: Incorporate controlled movements that gradually increase range of motion and warm up muscles, such as leg swings, arm circles, and walking lunges.
- **Yoga and Pilates**: Both practices combine stretching, strength, and mindfulness. Yoga emphasizes holding poses to improve flexibility and balance, while Pilates focuses on core strength and controlled movements.
- **Foam Rolling**: Use a foam roller to release muscle tightness (myofascial release), targeting areas of tension and promoting blood flow to muscles.

Effective Flexibility and Mobility Exercises

Hamstring Stretch:

Instructions: Sit on the floor with one leg extended straight and the other leg bent. Reach towards the extended leg's foot or ankle, keeping your back straight. Hold for 15-30 seconds and switch sides.

Quadriceps Stretch:

Instructions: Stand tall, balancing on one leg. Grab the ankle of your other leg and pull your heel towards your buttock. Keep knees close together and hold for 15-30 seconds. Switch sides.

Calf Stretch:

Instructions: Stand facing a wall with one foot forward and one foot back, both feet flat on the ground. Lean forward, keeping your back leg straight and heel on the floor, until you feel a stretch in your calf. Hold for 15-30 seconds and switch legs.

Child's Pose (Yoga):

Instructions: Kneel on the floor, sitting back on your heels. Extend your arms forward, lowering your chest towards the floor and resting your forehead on the ground. Hold for 15-30 seconds, focusing on deep breathing.

Cat-Cow Stretch (Yoga):

Instructions: Start on your hands and knees, with wrists aligned under shoulders and knees under hips. Inhale as you arch your back, dropping your belly towards the floor (Cow Pose). Exhale as you round your spine towards the ceiling, tucking your chin to your chest (Cat Pose). Repeat for 5-10 rounds.

Tips for Safe and Effective Stretching

- **Warm Up First**: Perform a light warm-up (e.g., brisk walking or jogging) before stretching to increase blood flow and prepare muscles for deeper stretches.

- **Focus on Breathing**: Breathe deeply and steadily during stretches to enhance relaxation and facilitate muscle relaxation.
- **Avoid Bouncing**: Perform stretches slowly and smoothly without bouncing, which can cause muscle strain or injury.
- **Stretch Both Sides**: Always stretch your body evenly to maintain balance and symmetry.
- **Be Consistent**: Incorporate flexibility and mobility exercises into your routine at least 2-3 times per week to maintain and improve your range of motion over time.

Flexibility and mobility exercises are integral to women's fitness routines, promoting improved range of motion, reduced muscle tension, enhanced athletic performance, and injury prevention. Incorporating stretching, yoga, Pilates, and other flexibility techniques into your workouts can enhance overall physical well-being and enjoy greater flexibility and mobility in daily activities. In the next chapter, we will discuss strategies for maintaining motivation, overcoming common fitness barriers, and integrating these exercises into a holistic approach to women's fitness.

3.4 Creating a Sustainable Workout Routine

Establishing a sustainable workout routine is crucial for achieving long-term fitness goals and maintaining overall health and well-being. This section explores strategies and considerations for creating a balanced and effective workout routine that you can maintain over time.

Key Considerations for a Sustainable Workout Routine

1. Set Realistic Goals:

Define clear and achievable fitness goals based on your current fitness level, interests, and lifestyle. Whether it's weight loss, muscle gain, improved flexibility, or overall health, setting specific goals helps you stay motivated and focused.

2. Assess Your Schedule and Commitment:

Evaluate your weekly schedule and identify the best times for exercise. Choose realistic workout durations and frequencies that fit into your routine without causing undue stress or fatigue.

3. Balance Cardiovascular, Strength, and Flexibility Training:

- Incorporate a variety of exercises to target different aspects of fitness:
  - **Cardiovascular Training**: Aim for 150 minutes of moderate-intensity aerobic exercise or 75 minutes of vigorous-intensity exercise per week, spread across most days.
  - **Strength Training**: Include sessions 2-3 times per week, focusing on major muscle groups with resistance exercises.
  - **Flexibility and Mobility**: Dedicate time for stretching, yoga, or Pilates exercises to improve flexibility and prevent injury.

4. Progression and Variety:

Gradually increase the intensity, duration, or complexity of your workouts to continually challenge your body and prevent plateauing. Incorporate different exercises, techniques, or classes to keep your routine engaging and enjoyable.

5. Listen to Your Body:

Pay attention to how your body responds to exercise. Adjust your routine as needed to accommodate fatigue, soreness, or changes in fitness level. Rest and recovery are essential components of a sustainable workout routine.

6. Nutrition and Hydration:

Support your workouts with a balanced diet rich in nutrients and adequate hydration. Fuel your body before and after exercise to optimize performance and recovery.

Tips for Creating Your Workout Routine

1. Schedule Regular Exercise Sessions:

Block out dedicated times for workouts in your weekly calendar. Treat these appointments as non-negotiable commitments to prioritize your health and fitness.

2. Start with a Warm-Up and End with a Cool-Down:

Begin each workout with a 5-10 minute warm-up to prepare your muscles and joints. End with a 5-10 minute cool-down to lower heart rate, stretch muscles, and promote recovery.

3. Mix Up Your Workouts:

Include a variety of activities and exercises to prevent boredom and engage different muscle groups. This could include outdoor activities, group classes, home workouts, or gym sessions.

4. Track Your Progress:

Monitor your fitness progress by tracking workouts, recording measurements, or keeping a fitness journal. Celebrate achievements and milestones to stay motivated and committed to your routine.

5. Adapt to Life Changes:

Be flexible and adaptable in adjusting your workout routine to accommodate changes in schedule, travel, or personal commitments. Find creative ways to stay active even during busy times.

Overcoming Barriers to Consistency

- **Time Constraints**: Prioritize short, effective workouts or break longer sessions into smaller segments throughout the day.
- **Lack of Motivation**: Find workout activities that you enjoy and look forward to. Join fitness communities or work out with a friend to stay accountable and motivated.
- **Injury or Health Concerns**: Consult with a healthcare professional or fitness trainer for guidance on safe exercises and modifications to prevent or recover from injuries.
- **Environmental Factors**: Have alternative workout options for different weather conditions or consider indoor activities during extreme weather.
- **Mindset and Self-Care**: Practice self-compassion and mindfulness. Stay positive and patient with yourself as you progress towards your fitness goals.

Creating a sustainable workout routine involves planning, consistency, and a balanced approach to cardiovascular, strength, and flexibility training. By setting realistic goals, prioritizing regular exercise, and adapting to your body's needs and life circumstances, you can establish a routine that supports long-term health, fitness, and well-being. Incorporate these strategies into your lifestyle to enjoy the benefits of a healthy and active lifestyle for years to come.

3.5 Home Workouts vs. Gym Workouts

Choosing between home workouts and gym workouts is a personal decision that depends on individual preferences, goals, and lifestyle factors. This section compares the benefits and considerations of both options to help you decide which approach best suits your fitness needs.

Home Workouts

Benefits:

- **Convenience**: Work out from the comfort of your home, saving time on commuting to a gym.
- **Cost-Effective**: Avoid gym membership fees and save money on travel expenses.
- **Flexibility**: Schedule workouts at any time that fits your daily routine without being restricted by gym hours.
- **Privacy**: Enjoy a private setting where you can exercise without feeling self-conscious.
- **Accessibility**: Access to a variety of online workout programs, videos, and apps that cater to different fitness levels and goals.

Considerations:

- **Limited Equipment**: Depending on your setup, home workouts may require investing in basic equipment such as dumbbells, resistance bands, or a yoga mat.

- **Space Requirements**: You need sufficient space to move comfortably and safely during exercises, which can be challenging in smaller living areas.
- **Motivation**: Staying motivated without the social atmosphere, equipment variety, or guidance from fitness professionals found in gyms.
- **Distractions**: Potential interruptions from family members, pets, or household chores may affect focus during workouts.

Gym Workouts

Benefits:

- **Equipment Variety**: Access to a wide range of fitness equipment and machines that may not be available at home, allowing for more diverse workout options.
- **Social Atmosphere**: Opportunity to exercise alongside others, participate in group classes, or seek advice and support from fitness trainers or fellow gym members.
- **Motivation and Accountability**: Surrounding yourself with like-minded individuals and professional guidance can enhance motivation and accountability.
- **Structured Environment**: A dedicated space designed for fitness, providing a conducive environment for focused workouts.
- **Additional Amenities**: Some gyms offer amenities such as pools, saunas, and specialized classes that can enrich your fitness experience.

Considerations:

- **Cost**: Membership fees and potential additional costs for classes, personal training, or amenities.
- **Travel Time**: Commuting to and from the gym adds to your workout time and may be less convenient on busy days.
- **Crowds**: Popular gyms may be crowded during peak hours, leading to wait times for equipment or limited space for workouts.
- **Schedule Dependence**: Workouts must align with gym operating hours, limiting flexibility in scheduling.

Choosing the Right Option

- **Consider Your Goals**: Determine whether your fitness goals require specific equipment or professional guidance that is more readily available at a gym.
- **Evaluate Lifestyle**: Assess factors such as time constraints, budget, motivation preferences, and access to space and equipment at home.
- **Mix and Match**: You can combine both approaches by using home workouts for convenience and gym sessions for a variety of specialized training needs.
- **Trial Period**: Try different options to see which environment motivates you the most and helps you achieve your fitness goals effectively.

Whether you choose home workouts or gym workouts, both options offer unique benefits and considerations that cater to different preferences and fitness objectives. The key is to select an approach that aligns with your lifestyle, motivates you to stay consistent, and supports your journey toward improved health and fitness. By understanding the pros and cons of each option, you can make an informed decision that enhances your overall fitness experience and enjoyment.

Chapter 4: Lifestyle and Behavioral Changes

In the pursuit of achieving sustainable weight loss and overall health improvement, embracing lifestyle and behavioral changes is pivotal. This chapter explores the essential aspects of transforming habits, mindset shifts, and strategies for overcoming challenges on the path to long-term wellness.

Understanding Behavioral Change

Behavioral change involves adopting new habits and modifying existing behaviors to foster healthier choices and achieve fitness goals. It requires understanding the psychological factors influencing our actions and implementing strategies that promote lasting change. By recognizing the importance of behavioral change, individuals can empower themselves to make positive shifts in their lifestyles.

Embracing Mindset Shifts

A fundamental aspect of successful lifestyle change is cultivating a positive mindset. This begins with self-compassion, replacing self-criticism with understanding and kindness towards oneself. Setting SMART goals—specific, measurable, achievable, relevant, and time-bound—provides clarity and direction. Celebrating progress, no matter how small, fosters motivation and resilience in the face of setbacks. Embracing setbacks as opportunities for growth and maintaining a steadfast commitment to long-term goals are essential components of a resilient mindset.

Strategies for Habit Formation

Building sustainable habits involves starting small and gradually integrating new behaviors into daily routines. Consistency is key, as repeated actions reinforce neural pathways and make habits automatic. Environment design plays a crucial role; arranging surroundings to support healthy choices—such as keeping nutritious foods visible and accessible—encourages adherence to new habits. Behavioral cues, like setting reminders or establishing a regular workout schedule, serve as prompts for desired actions, aiding in habit formation.

Nutrition and Eating Behaviors

A balanced diet forms the cornerstone of overall health and weight management. Practicing mindful eating—paying attention to hunger cues, savoring food, and avoiding distractions—supports healthy eating behaviors. Portion control, understanding appropriate serving sizes, and mindful consumption of nutrients contribute to maintaining a healthy caloric balance.

Integrating Physical Activity

Regular exercise is essential for achieving and maintaining physical fitness. Incorporating diverse forms of exercise—cardiovascular, strength training, and flexibility exercises—supports holistic health benefits. Embracing an active lifestyle involves seeking opportunities for movement throughout the day, such as walking or biking instead of driving, taking stairs instead of elevators, and participating in recreational activities.

Stress Management and Sleep

Effective stress management techniques—such as deep breathing, meditation, yoga, or engaging in hobbies—promote relaxation and reduce stress levels. Quality sleep is crucial for overall health, energy restoration, and recovery from physical activity. Prioritizing sufficient sleep supports optimal cognitive function, mood regulation, and physical well-being.

Cultivating Social Support and Accountability

Engaging with a supportive social network—friends, family, or fitness communities—encourages and reinforces commitment to health goals. Accountability partners, such as workout buddies or fitness coaches, offer guidance, motivation, and accountability in maintaining a consistent fitness regimen.

Overcoming Challenges

Identifying triggers that may hinder progress and developing strategies to manage them effectively are essential for overcoming challenges. Learning from setbacks—viewing them as temporary and adjusting approaches accordingly—strengthens resilience and promotes continued growth towards achieving health goals.

Incorporating lifestyle and behavioral changes is fundamental to achieving sustainable weight loss, enhancing overall health, and cultivating a fulfilling life. By adopting a positive mindset, implementing effective strategies for habit formation, prioritizing nutrition and physical activity, managing stress, fostering social support, and learning from challenges, individuals can establish a foundation for lasting wellness. This chapter provides actionable insights and guidance to empower individuals in making meaningful lifestyle changes and navigating their journey towards optimal health and well-being.

4.1 Building Healthy Habits

Building healthy habits is integral to achieving sustainable lifestyle changes that support overall health and well-being. It involves adopting behaviors that contribute positively to your physical, mental, and emotional wellness. Here's how to effectively build and maintain healthy habits:

Starting Small

Begin by focusing on small, achievable changes that align with your goals. Starting small increases the likelihood of success and reduces the feeling of overwhelm. For example, if your goal is to drink more water, start by replacing one sugary drink with a glass of water each day.

Consistency is Key

Consistently practicing new behaviors reinforces habits over time. Aim to incorporate your chosen habit into your daily routine. Whether it's exercising, preparing healthy meals, or practicing mindfulness, commit to regular and consistent efforts to solidify the habit.

Setting Clear Goals

Set clear and specific goals to guide your habit-building process. Use the SMART criteria—Specific, Measurable, Achievable, Relevant, and Time-bound—to define your objectives. For instance, if you aim to exercise more, set a goal to walk for 30 minutes five days a week.

Environment and Cue Management

Modify your environment to support your desired habits. Make healthy choices more accessible and convenient. For instance, keep fruits and vegetables visible and reachable in your kitchen. Use cues or reminders—such as alarms or calendar alerts—to prompt your desired behavior.

Accountability and Support

Engage with others who share similar goals or seek support from friends, family, or online communities. Accountability partners can provide encouragement, motivation, and feedback, enhancing your commitment to building and maintaining healthy habits.

Tracking Progress and Celebrating Success

Monitor your progress regularly to stay motivated and identify areas for improvement. Keep a journal, use a habit-tracking app, or create a checklist to record your daily efforts. Celebrate milestones and successes along the way to reinforce positive behaviors.

Overcoming Setbacks and Staying Resilient

Accept that setbacks are a natural part of behavior change. Learn from setbacks by identifying triggers or obstacles that hinder your progress. Develop strategies to overcome challenges and adapt your approach as needed. Cultivating resilience and staying committed to your goals will help you navigate through setbacks and continue on your path to building healthy habits.

Building healthy habits requires dedication, consistency, and a proactive approach to behavior change. By starting small, setting clear goals, managing your environment and cues, seeking support and accountability, tracking progress, and staying resilient in the face of challenges, you can establish lasting habits that promote overall health and well-being. Incorporate these strategies into your daily life to cultivate positive behaviors that contribute to a healthier and more fulfilling lifestyle.

4.2 Overcoming Emotional Eating

Emotional eating is a common behavior where individuals use food as a means to cope with emotions, such as stress, sadness, boredom, or even happiness. It often involves consuming larger amounts of food than necessary, leading to feelings of guilt and undermining health and weight management goals. Overcoming emotional eating requires awareness, understanding triggers, and developing alternative coping strategies.

Recognizing Emotional Eating

Identifying emotional eating involves becoming aware of the patterns and situations in which you turn to food for emotional comfort rather than physical hunger. Common signs include eating when not physically hungry, eating to numb emotions or distract from feelings, and experiencing guilt or regret after eating.

Understanding Triggers

Emotional eating is often triggered by emotional states, such as stress, loneliness, boredom, anxiety, or even happiness. It can also be triggered by environmental cues, such as seeing food advertisements or passing by a favorite restaurant. Recognizing your specific triggers helps you anticipate situations where emotional eating may occur.

Strategies to Overcome Emotional Eating

- **Mindful Eating**: Practice mindfulness techniques to become more aware of your eating habits and emotional triggers. Pause before eating to assess your hunger level and emotional state. Eat slowly, savoring each bite, and pay attention to how different foods make you feel.

- **Find Alternative Coping Mechanisms**: Develop healthier ways to manage emotions instead of turning to food. Engage in activities that provide comfort or relaxation, such as going for a walk, practicing yoga, journaling, talking to a friend, or listening to music.
- **Manage Stress Effectively**: Implement stress-reduction techniques, such as deep breathing, meditation, or progressive muscle relaxation, to reduce the urge to eat in response to stress.
- **Create a Supportive Environment**: Surround yourself with supportive friends, family, or a therapist who can offer encouragement and help you navigate emotional challenges without relying on food.
- **Healthy Lifestyle Habits**: Establish regular eating patterns with balanced meals and snacks throughout the day to maintain stable blood sugar levels and reduce the likelihood of emotional eating episodes.
- **Limit Access to Trigger Foods**: If certain foods consistently trigger emotional eating, consider reducing their availability or finding healthier alternatives that satisfy cravings without compromising your goals.

Breaking the Cycle

Breaking the cycle of emotional eating involves changing your relationship with food and developing healthier coping mechanisms for managing emotions. It requires patience, self-awareness, and a commitment to practicing alternative strategies over time.

Seeking Professional Help

If emotional eating significantly impacts your well-being or if you find it challenging to overcome on your own, consider seeking support from a registered dietitian, therapist, or counselor specializing in eating behaviors. They can provide personalized strategies and support to address underlying emotional triggers and develop a healthier relationship with food.

Overcoming emotional eating is a journey that begins with self-awareness and involves developing alternative coping strategies, managing triggers, and fostering a supportive environment. By practicing mindfulness, finding healthy outlets for emotions, managing stress effectively, and seeking professional guidance when needed, you can break free from emotional eating patterns and cultivate a balanced approach to eating that supports your overall health and well-being.

4.3 Stress Management Techniques

Effective stress management is essential for maintaining overall well-being and improving health outcomes. Stress, if left unchecked, can negatively impact physical health, mental clarity, and emotional stability. This section explores various techniques and strategies to help manage and reduce stress in daily life.

Deep Breathing Exercises

Deep breathing exercises, such as diaphragmatic breathing or belly breathing, promote relaxation and reduce stress. Focus on taking slow, deep breaths, inhaling through your nose, and exhaling through your mouth. Deep breathing increases oxygen flow, slows your heart rate, and calms your mind.

Progressive Muscle Relaxation (PMR)

Progressive Muscle Relaxation involves tensing and then relaxing different muscle groups throughout your body. Start by tensing muscles for a few seconds, then release and relax them completely. This technique helps relieve physical tension and promotes a sense of relaxation.

Mindfulness Meditation

Mindfulness meditation involves focusing your attention on the present moment without judgment. Find a quiet place, sit comfortably, and concentrate on your breath or a specific sensation. Mindfulness meditation reduces stress by promoting relaxation, enhancing self-awareness, and fostering a sense of calm.

Exercise and Physical Activity

Engaging in regular physical activity, such as walking, jogging, yoga, or dancing, reduces stress hormones like cortisol and releases endorphins that improve mood. Exercise also promotes better sleep, boosts self-esteem, and provides a healthy outlet for stress.

Time Management and Prioritization

Effective time management helps reduce stress by organizing tasks and responsibilities. Prioritize tasks based on urgency and importance, break large tasks into smaller ones, and set realistic deadlines. Create a daily or weekly schedule to manage time efficiently and reduce feelings of overwhelm.

Relaxation Techniques

Explore relaxation techniques that suit your preferences, such as listening to calming music, taking a warm bath, practicing yoga or tai chi, or engaging in hobbies like painting or gardening. Relaxation techniques promote relaxation, reduce muscle tension, and alleviate stress.

Social Support and Connection

Maintain supportive relationships with friends, family, or peers who offer encouragement and understanding during stressful times. Connect with others through social activities, join clubs or groups with shared interests, and seek emotional support when needed.

Healthy Lifestyle Choices

Adopting a healthy lifestyle supports stress management. Eat a balanced diet rich in fruits, vegetables, lean proteins, and whole grains to support overall health. Limit caffeine and alcohol intake, which can exacerbate stress and anxiety. Prioritize sufficient sleep to restore energy levels and enhance resilience to stress.

Cognitive Behavioral Techniques (CBT)

Cognitive Behavioral Therapy techniques help identify and change negative thought patterns and behaviors that contribute to stress. Practice reframing negative thoughts into more positive or realistic perspectives. CBT promotes adaptive coping strategies and reduces stress-related symptoms.

Seeking Professional Help

If stress becomes overwhelming or persistent, seek support from a mental health professional, counselor, or therapist. They can provide personalized strategies, tools, and therapeutic interventions to manage stress effectively and improve overall well-being.

Incorporating stress management techniques into your daily routine promotes resilience, enhances coping skills, and improves overall quality of life. By practicing deep breathing exercises, progressive muscle relaxation, mindfulness meditation, regular exercise, effective time management, relaxation techniques, maintaining social connections, making healthy lifestyle choices, utilizing cognitive behavioral techniques, and seeking professional help when needed, you can effectively manage stress and foster a sense of calm and balance in your life.

4.4 The Role of Sleep in Weight Loss

Sleep plays a crucial role in overall health and well-being, including its impact on weight management and metabolism. Understanding how sleep influences weight loss efforts is essential for achieving sustainable results and improving overall health outcomes.

Sleep Duration and Quality

Both the duration and quality of sleep significantly affect various physiological processes related to weight regulation. Adults typically require 7-9 hours of sleep per night for optimal health. Poor sleep quality, characterized by frequent awakenings or disruptions, can impair metabolic function and contribute to weight gain.

Hormonal Regulation

Sleep influences the production and balance of hormones that regulate appetite, hunger, and satiety. Inadequate sleep disrupts the hormonal balance, increasing levels of ghrelin (hunger hormone) and decreasing levels of leptin (satiety hormone). This hormonal imbalance can lead to increased appetite, cravings for high-calorie foods, and overeating, ultimately contributing to weight gain.

Metabolic Function

Quality sleep is crucial for maintaining proper metabolic function. Sleep deprivation alters glucose metabolism and insulin sensitivity, leading to impaired glucose tolerance and increased risk of developing insulin resistance. These metabolic changes can hinder weight loss efforts and promote fat storage.

Energy Balance and Food Choices

Sleep deprivation affects decision-making processes related to food choices and energy balance. Individuals experiencing sleep deprivation are more likely to choose high-calorie, sugary, and fatty foods over healthier options. These poor food choices can disrupt energy balance, increase caloric intake, and contribute to weight gain over time.

Physical Activity and Exercise Performance

Adequate sleep supports physical performance and exercise recovery. Sleep deprivation impairs motor skills, coordination, and reaction times, reducing the quality and intensity of physical activity. Furthermore, insufficient sleep compromises muscle recovery and repair, limiting the benefits of exercise for weight loss and muscle development.

Psychological Well-being and Stress Management

Quality sleep promotes emotional resilience and mental clarity, which are crucial for managing stress and emotional eating behaviors. Sleep deprivation increases stress levels and disrupts emotional regulation, leading to heightened cortisol levels (stress hormone) that can contribute to abdominal fat accumulation and weight gain.

Strategies for Improving Sleep Quality

- **Establish a Sleep Routine**: Maintain consistent sleep and wake times, even on weekends, to regulate your body's internal clock.
- **Create a Restful Environment**: Design a sleep-friendly environment by reducing noise, controlling room temperature, and ensuring comfort with a supportive mattress and pillows.
- **Limit Stimulants and Screen Time**: Avoid caffeine and heavy meals before bedtime, and minimize exposure to screens (e.g., phones, computers) that emit blue light, which can disrupt sleep patterns.
- **Practice Relaxation Techniques**: Engage in relaxation practices such as deep breathing, meditation, or gentle yoga before bed to promote relaxation and prepare your mind for sleep.
- **Address Sleep Disorders**: If you suspect sleep disorders like sleep apnea or insomnia, seek evaluation and treatment from a healthcare professional to improve sleep quality and overall health.

Quality sleep is a critical component of successful weight management and overall health. By prioritizing sufficient and restorative sleep, individuals can support hormonal balance, enhance metabolic function, improve food choices, optimize physical performance, manage stress effectively, and promote overall well-being. Incorporating strategies to improve sleep quality alongside healthy diet and exercise habits is essential for achieving sustainable weight loss and maintaining long-term health outcomes.

4.5 Staying Motivated and Consistent

Maintaining motivation and consistency are key factors in achieving long-term success in weight loss and overall health improvement. These qualities help individuals overcome challenges, stay committed to their goals, and sustain positive lifestyle changes over time.

Setting Clear Goals

Begin by establishing clear and realistic goals that provide direction and motivation. Use the SMART criteria—Specific, Measurable, Achievable, Relevant, and Time-bound—to define your objectives. Clear goals help clarify your purpose and enable you to track progress effectively.

Finding Your Motivation

Identify your reasons for wanting to achieve weight loss and improved health. Whether it's enhancing self-esteem, improving energy levels, or reducing health risks, understanding your motivation strengthens your commitment and resilience during challenging times.

Developing Healthy Habits

Focus on building sustainable habits that support your health goals. Start with small, manageable changes and gradually incorporate them into your daily routine. Consistency in practicing healthy behaviors, such as regular exercise and balanced nutrition, reinforces positive habits over time.

Celebrating Progress

Acknowledge and celebrate your achievements, no matter how small. Recognizing milestones along the way boosts motivation and reinforces your commitment to continued progress. Celebrate achievements with non-food rewards that align with your health goals, such as treating yourself to a spa day or buying new workout gear.

Seeking Support and Accountability

Engage with a support system of friends, family, or a community who share similar health goals. Accountability partners can provide encouragement, share experiences, and offer valuable support during challenging moments. Consider joining group fitness classes, or online forums, or seeking guidance from a healthcare professional or certified coach.

Embracing Positive Self-Talk

Practice positive self-talk and cultivate a mindset of self-compassion. Replace self-criticism with supportive and encouraging thoughts. Focus on your strengths and progress, learning from setbacks as opportunities for growth rather than reasons for discouragement.

Adjusting Your Approach

Be flexible and willing to adjust your approach as needed. Recognize that setbacks are a natural part of the journey and use them as learning opportunities. Evaluate what works well and what can be improved, then make necessary adjustments to stay on track towards your goals.

Creating a Supportive Environment

Surround yourself with a supportive environment that fosters healthy behaviors. Arrange your surroundings to promote positive choices, such as keeping healthy snacks readily available and creating a dedicated space for exercise. Minimize temptations and distractions that may hinder your progress.

Practicing Patience and Persistence

Understand that sustainable change takes time and requires patience. Stay focused on the long-term benefits of improved health and well-being. Stay persistent in your efforts, even during periods of slow progress or temporary setbacks.

Staying motivated and consistent is essential for achieving and maintaining weight loss and overall health improvement. By setting clear goals, finding intrinsic motivation, developing healthy habits, celebrating progress, seeking support, embracing positive self-talk, adjusting your approach, creating a supportive environment, and practicing patience and persistence, you can cultivate a mindset and lifestyle that supports long-term success.

Chapter 5: Understanding and Using Supplements

Supplements play a significant role in many individuals' health and fitness routines, offering a convenient way to support nutritional needs and enhance overall well-being. This chapter explores the fundamentals of supplements, including their benefits, considerations for use, and how to integrate them effectively into a balanced lifestyle.

Introduction to Supplements

Supplements are products designed to supplement the diet with nutrients that may be lacking or insufficiently consumed through food alone. They come in various forms, including vitamins, minerals, herbal extracts, amino acids, and other substances intended to support health and wellness.

Benefits of Supplements

- **Nutritional Support**: Supplements can provide essential vitamins and minerals that support overall health and fill nutritional gaps in the diet.
- **Enhanced Performance**: Certain supplements, such as those used by athletes, may enhance physical performance, endurance, and recovery.
- **Convenience**: They offer a convenient way to ensure consistent intake of specific nutrients, especially for individuals with busy lifestyles or dietary restrictions.

- **Targeted Health Goals**: Supplements can be tailored to support specific health goals, such as weight management, immune support, or joint health.

Types of Supplements

- **Vitamins and Minerals**: Essential nutrients that support various bodily functions, including vitamin C, vitamin D, calcium, and iron.
- **Herbal Supplements**: Derived from plants and used for various purposes, such as improving immunity, reducing inflammation, or promoting relaxation.
- **Protein Supplements**: Including whey protein, casein, and plant-based proteins, which support muscle growth and recovery.
- **Omega-3 Fatty Acids**: Found in fish oil supplements, omega-3s support heart health, brain function, and inflammation reduction.
- **Sports and Performance Supplements**: Including creatine, caffeine, and BCAAs (branched-chain amino acids), which are used to enhance athletic performance and recovery.

Considerations for Use

- **Consultation with Healthcare Providers**: Before starting any supplement regimen, consult with a healthcare provider, especially if you have underlying health conditions or are taking medications.
- **Quality and Safety**: Choose supplements from reputable brands that adhere to quality standards and are certified by regulatory authorities (e.g., FDA, NSF).

- **Dosage and Timing**: Follow recommended dosages provided by manufacturers and consider the best timing for ingestion to optimize absorption and effectiveness.
- **Potential Interactions**: Be aware of potential interactions between supplements and medications or other supplements you may be taking. Certain combinations can affect absorption or efficacy.

Integrating Supplements into Your Routine

- **Assess Nutritional Needs**: Identify any nutrient deficiencies or areas where your diet may fall short, then select supplements to address those needs.
- **Start Gradually**: Introduce supplements gradually into your routine to monitor for any adverse reactions or changes in health.
- **Monitor Effects**: Pay attention to how supplements affect your body and overall well-being. Adjust dosage or discontinue use if you experience negative side effects.
- **Combined with Healthy Lifestyle**: Supplements are most effective when combined with a balanced diet, regular physical activity, adequate sleep, and stress management practices.

Understanding supplements empowers individuals to make informed decisions about their health and wellness. By recognizing the benefits of supplements, understanding different types, considering proper use and safety guidelines, and integrating them into a holistic approach to health, individuals can optimize their nutritional intake and support their overall well-being effectively. This chapter provides a foundational understanding of supplements, guiding readers toward making educated choices that align with their health goals and lifestyle preferences.

5.1 Overview of Popular Supplements

Supplements are widely used to support health and wellness goals, offering targeted nutrients that may be lacking in the diet or needed in higher amounts for specific purposes. Understanding the most popular types of supplements provides insight into their benefits and considerations for use.

Multivitamins

Multivitamins are comprehensive supplements that contain a combination of vitamins and minerals essential for overall health. They are designed to fill nutritional gaps in the diet and support general well-being. Multivitamins typically include vitamins A, C, D, E, K, and B vitamins, and minerals like calcium, magnesium, zinc, and iron.

Omega-3 Fatty Acids

Omega-3 fatty acids, found in fish oil supplements, are renowned for their health benefits, particularly for heart health and brain function. They include EPA (eicosapentaenoic acid) and DHA (docosahexaenoic acid), essential fatty acids that are important for reducing inflammation, supporting cardiovascular health, and promoting cognitive function.

Vitamin D

Vitamin D supplements are crucial for maintaining optimal bone health and supporting immune function. Often referred to as the "sunshine vitamin," vitamin D is synthesized in the skin in response to sunlight exposure. Supplementing with vitamin D is recommended, especially for individuals who have limited sun exposure or live in regions with inadequate sunlight during certain seasons.

Probiotics

Probiotics are beneficial bacteria that promote a healthy balance of gut microflora. These supplements support digestive health, improve immune function, and may even enhance mood and cognitive function. Probiotics are commonly found in fermented foods like yogurt, kefir, and sauerkraut, as well as in supplement form with specific strains such as Lactobacillus and Bifidobacterium.

Protein Supplements

Protein supplements, including whey protein, casein, and plant-based proteins (e.g., soy, pea, hemp), are popular among athletes and individuals seeking to support muscle growth, recovery, and overall protein intake. These supplements are convenient for post-workout nutrition or as meal replacements and come in various forms, including powders, bars, and ready-to-drink shakes.

Calcium

Calcium supplements are essential for maintaining strong bones and teeth. Adequate calcium intake is crucial throughout life, particularly during adolescence and older adulthood when bone density declines. Calcium supplements are available in various forms, such as calcium carbonate and calcium citrate, and are often combined with vitamin D for better absorption.

Herbal Supplements

Herbal supplements derive from plants and are used for various health purposes. Examples include ginkgo biloba for cognitive function, turmeric for anti-inflammatory effects, echinacea for immune support, and St. John's wort for mood enhancement. Herbal supplements should be used with caution, as they can interact with medications and vary in potency and purity.

Considerations for Use

When considering supplements, it's essential to:

- **Consult Healthcare Providers**: Discuss supplement use with healthcare providers, especially if you have underlying health conditions or take medications.
- **Quality and Safety**: Choose supplements from reputable brands that undergo third-party testing and adhere to quality standards.
- **Dosage and Timing**: Follow recommended dosages provided by manufacturers and consider the best timing for ingestion to optimize absorption and effectiveness.

- **Monitor Effects**: Pay attention to how supplements affect your body and overall well-being. Adjust dosage or discontinue use if you experience adverse effects.

Understanding the overview of popular supplements empowers individuals to make informed decisions about their health and well-being. Whether addressing specific nutrient deficiencies, supporting athletic performance, or enhancing overall vitality, supplements can complement a balanced diet and lifestyle. By considering benefits, safety considerations, and proper integration into daily routines, individuals can optimize their health goals effectively with the use of supplements.

5.2 Benefits and Risks of Supplements

Supplements offer various benefits in supporting health and wellness goals, but they also come with considerations regarding potential risks and side effects. Understanding both aspects is essential for making informed decisions about supplement use.

Benefits of Supplements

- **Nutritional Support**: Supplements provide essential vitamins, minerals, and nutrients that may be lacking in the diet, helping to fill nutritional gaps and support overall health.
- **Convenience**: They offer a convenient way to ensure consistent intake of specific nutrients, especially for individuals with dietary restrictions, busy lifestyles, or inadequate nutrient intake from food alone.

- **Targeted Health Goals**: Certain supplements are designed to support specific health goals, such as immune support, joint health, cognitive function, or athletic performance.
- **Improved Bone Health**: Supplements like calcium and vitamin D support bone strength and density, reducing the risk of osteoporosis and fractures, particularly in older adults.
- **Enhanced Athletic Performance**: Supplements such as protein, creatine, and branched-chain amino acids (BCAAs) can enhance muscle growth, strength, endurance, and recovery in athletes and active individuals.
- **Heart Health**: Omega-3 fatty acids (found in fish oil supplements) support cardiovascular health by reducing inflammation, lowering triglyceride levels, and improving cholesterol profiles.

Risks and Considerations

- **Potential for Toxicity**: Overconsumption of certain vitamins and minerals, particularly fat-soluble vitamins (e.g., vitamin A, vitamin D), can lead to toxicity and adverse health effects.
- **Interactions with Medications**: Supplements can interact with prescription medications, altering their effectiveness or causing unintended side effects. It's crucial to consult with healthcare providers before starting supplements, especially if taking medications.
- **Quality and Purity Concerns**: Supplements are not regulated as strictly as pharmaceutical drugs. Some products may contain contaminants, inconsistent potency, or misleading labeling claims. Choose supplements from reputable brands that adhere to quality standards and undergo third-party testing.

- **Digestive Upset**: Certain supplements, such as high doses of iron or magnesium, can cause gastrointestinal discomfort, including nausea, diarrhea, or constipation.
- **Allergic Reactions**: Individuals with allergies or sensitivities may experience allergic reactions to ingredients in supplements, including common allergens like soy, dairy, or gluten.
- **Long-Term Safety Data**: Limited research exists on the long-term safety and efficacy of many supplements, especially when used in high doses or over extended periods.

Guidelines for Safe Use

- **Consult Healthcare Providers**: Before starting any new supplement regimen, consult with a healthcare provider, particularly if you have underlying health conditions, are pregnant or breastfeeding, or take medications.
- **Follow Recommended Dosages**: Adhere to recommended dosages provided by manufacturers. Avoid exceeding recommended intake levels unless under the guidance of a healthcare provider.
- **Monitor for Side Effects**: Pay attention to how supplements affect your body. Discontinue use and seek medical advice if you experience adverse reactions or symptoms.
- **Choose Reputable Brands**: Select supplements from reputable brands that undergo third-party testing for quality, purity, and potency. Look for certifications from organizations like NSF International or USP (United States Pharmacopeia).
- **Integrate with Balanced Diet**: Supplements should complement, not replace, a balanced diet rich in whole foods. Focus on consuming nutrient-dense foods to meet most of your nutritional needs.

Supplements can be valuable tools for supporting health goals and addressing specific nutritional needs. However, it's essential to weigh the potential benefits against the risks and considerations associated with supplement use. By understanding the benefits, being aware of potential risks, following safety guidelines, and consulting healthcare providers when needed, individuals can make informed decisions to optimize their health and well-being effectively with supplements.

5.3 How to Choose the Right Supplements

Choosing the right supplements involves careful consideration of your individual health needs, the quality of the supplement, and safety aspects. Here are essential factors to help you make informed decisions:

1.   **Assess Your Nutritional Needs**

Evaluate your diet and identify any specific nutrients that may be lacking or insufficiently consumed. Consider factors such as age, gender, health conditions, dietary restrictions, and lifestyle habits that may affect your nutrient intake.

2.   **Identify Your Health Goals**

Determine your primary health goals or reasons for considering supplements. Whether you're aiming to support overall health, enhance athletic performance, manage specific health conditions, or address nutritional deficiencies, your goals will guide the selection of appropriate supplements.

3. Consult with Healthcare Providers

Before starting any new supplement regimen, consult with a healthcare provider, such as a registered dietitian, nutritionist, or physician. They can provide personalized recommendations based on your individual health status, medical history, medications, and specific health goals.

4. Research and Quality Assurance

Choose supplements from reputable brands that adhere to strict quality standards and undergo third-party testing for purity, potency, and safety. Look for certifications from organizations like NSF International, USP (United States Pharmacopeia), or ConsumerLab.com, which verify product quality.

5. Read Labels and Ingredients

Carefully read supplement labels to understand the ingredients, dosage recommendations, and any additional ingredients or allergens. Avoid supplements with unnecessary fillers, additives, or proprietary blends that may not disclose specific ingredient amounts.

6. Consider Form and Bioavailability

Select supplements in forms that are well-absorbed and bioavailable for your body. For example, choose vitamin D3 over vitamin D2 for better absorption, or opt for chelated minerals (e.g., magnesium glycinate) for improved bioavailability compared to other forms.

7.   Avoid Excessive Claims and Misleading Information

Be cautious of supplements that make exaggerated claims or promise unrealistic outcomes. Look for evidence-based information supported by scientific research and clinical studies rather than marketing hype.

8.   Evaluate Cost and Value

Compare costs among different brands and products, considering factors like dosage, servings per container, and quality. While price is important, prioritize quality and effectiveness to ensure you're investing in supplements that support your health goals.

9.   Monitor and Adjust

Start with one supplement at a time, if possible, to monitor how your body responds. Pay attention to any changes in symptoms, side effects, or improvements in health. Adjust dosage or discontinue supplements if necessary, under the guidance of a healthcare provider.

10. Integrate with a Balanced Diet

Remember that supplements are meant to complement, not replace, a balanced diet rich in nutrient-dense foods. Focus on consuming a variety of fruits, vegetables, whole grains, lean proteins, and healthy fats to meet most of your nutritional needs.

Choosing the right supplements requires careful consideration of your individual health needs, goals, quality assurance, and safety aspects. By assessing your nutritional needs, consulting healthcare providers, researching reputable brands, reading labels, considering bioavailability, avoiding excessive claims, evaluating cost and value, monitoring effects, and integrating with a balanced diet, you can make informed decisions to support your health and well-being effectively with supplements. Always prioritize safety, quality, and evidence-based information when selecting supplements for your health regimen.

5.4 Integrating Supplements into Your Routine

Integrating supplements into your daily routine effectively involves thoughtful planning, consistency, and adherence to recommended guidelines. Whether you're new to supplement use or looking to optimize your regimen, consider the following steps for seamless integration:

1. Identify Specific Health Goals

Define your health goals and objectives that supplements can support. Whether you're aiming to enhance overall health, address specific deficiencies, support athletic performance, or manage health conditions, clear goals guide your supplement choices.

2. Consult with Healthcare Providers

Before starting any new supplements, consult with healthcare providers such as a registered dietitian, nutritionist, or physician. They can assess your health status, review your current medications, and provide personalized recommendations tailored to your needs.

3. Choose High-Quality Supplements

Select supplements from reputable brands that adhere to stringent quality standards and undergo third-party testing for purity, potency, and safety. Look for certifications from organizations like NSF International, USP (United States Pharmacopeia), or ConsumerLab.com to ensure product quality.

4. Follow Recommended Dosages

Adhere to recommended dosages provided by healthcare providers or as indicated on the supplement labels. Avoid exceeding recommended intake levels unless advised by a healthcare professional, as excessive intake can lead to adverse effects or toxicity.

5. Establish a Consistent Routine

Incorporate supplements into your daily routine at consistent times, such as with meals or as directed by healthcare providers. Establishing a routine helps ensure regular intake and supports optimal absorption of nutrients.

6. Consider Compatibility and Interactions

Be mindful of potential interactions between supplements and medications you may be taking. Certain supplements, such as calcium, iron, or vitamin K, can interfere with the absorption or effectiveness of medications. Discuss potential interactions with healthcare providers to minimize risks.

7. Monitor Effects and Adjust as Needed

Pay attention to how supplements affect your body and overall well-being. Monitor for any changes in symptoms, improvements in health outcomes, or potential side effects. Adjust supplement dosages or formulations based on feedback from healthcare providers.

8. Integrate with a Balanced Diet

Supplements are intended to complement, not replace, a balanced diet rich in nutrient-dense foods. Focus on consuming a variety of fruits, vegetables, whole grains, lean proteins, and healthy fats to meet most of your nutritional needs naturally.

9.   Maintain Transparency with Healthcare Providers

Keep healthcare providers informed about all supplements you are taking, including dosage and frequency. This transparency allows them to monitor your overall health status, assess any potential interactions, and make adjustments as needed.

10. Evaluate Long-Term Benefits

Regularly assess the long-term benefits of supplement use in achieving your health goals. Evaluate improvements in energy levels, immune function, athletic performance, or specific health conditions to determine the effectiveness of your supplement regimen.

Integrating supplements into your routine involves careful planning, adherence to recommended guidelines, and collaboration with healthcare providers. By identifying health goals, consulting with professionals, choosing high-quality supplements, following recommended dosages, establishing a consistent routine, considering interactions, monitoring effects, integrating with a balanced diet, maintaining transparency, and evaluating long-term benefits, you can effectively optimize your health regimen with supplements. Prioritize safety, quality, and consistency to support your journey toward improved health and well-being.

Chapter 6: Monitoring Progress and Adjusting Goals

Monitoring progress and adjusting goals are essential components of achieving long-term success in any health and fitness endeavor. This chapter explores effective strategies for tracking your progress, evaluating outcomes, and making necessary adjustments to your goals to maintain motivation and optimize results.

Setting Clear Metrics

Start by establishing clear metrics that align with your health and fitness goals. Whether you're aiming to lose weight, build muscle, improve cardiovascular fitness, or enhance overall well-being, defining specific, measurable objectives provides a benchmark for tracking progress.

Tracking Tools and Methods

Utilize various tracking tools and methods to monitor your progress effectively:

- **Measurement and Body Composition**: Track changes in weight, body fat percentage, and measurements (e.g., waist circumference, muscle mass).
- **Fitness Assessments**: Conduct periodic fitness assessments, such as cardiovascular endurance tests, strength evaluations (e.g., one-repetition maximum), and flexibility measurements.

- **Nutritional Logs**: Keep food journals or use mobile apps to monitor dietary intake, including calories, macronutrients (proteins, carbs, fats), and micronutrients.
- **Activity and Exercise Logs**: Record physical activity and exercise sessions, noting duration, intensity, and type of workouts performed.

Evaluating Outcomes

Regularly evaluate outcomes based on your tracked metrics and assessments:

- **Progress towards Goals**: Assess whether you're moving closer to achieving your initial objectives within the specified timeframe.
- **Adherence to Plan**: Review consistency in following your exercise regimen, dietary guidelines, and supplement routine.
- **Health Markers**: Consider improvements in health markers such as blood pressure, cholesterol levels, blood sugar levels, and overall energy levels.

Adjusting Goals and Strategies

Based on your evaluation, make adjustments to your goals and strategies as needed:

- **Modify Targets**: Adjust timelines, set new milestones, or refine specific targets to maintain motivation and progress.

- **Change Approaches**: Modify exercise routines, dietary plans, or supplement regimens to better align with your current needs and preferences.
- **Seek Expert Guidance**: Consult with healthcare providers, fitness trainers, or nutritionists for professional guidance and support in adjusting your goals and strategies.

Staying Motivated

Stay motivated throughout your journey by:

- **Celebrating Achievements**: Acknowledge and celebrate milestones and accomplishments, no matter how small.
- **Visualizing Success**: Visualize your long-term goals and the benefits of achieving them to stay focused and committed.
- **Seeking Support**: Engage with a supportive community, friends, or family members who encourage and motivate you.

Practicing Patience and Persistence

Recognize that progress takes time and requires consistent effort:

- **Stay Consistent**: Maintain consistency in your routines and habits, even during challenging periods.
- **Learn from Setbacks**: View setbacks as learning opportunities and adjust your approach accordingly.

Monitoring progress and adjusting goals are crucial aspects of achieving sustainable health and fitness outcomes. By setting clear metrics, utilizing tracking tools, evaluating outcomes, making necessary adjustments, staying motivated, practicing patience, and seeking support, you can effectively navigate your health journey. Continuously assess your progress, adapt strategies as needed, and celebrate your achievements along the way to maintain momentum and achieve long-term success in reaching your health and fitness goals.

6.1 Tracking Your Progress

Tracking your progress is essential for effectively monitoring your journey towards achieving health and fitness goals. By establishing clear metrics and utilizing various tracking methods, you can assess your advancements, identify areas for improvement, and stay motivated throughout your wellness journey.

Establish Clear Metrics

Start by defining specific and measurable metrics that align with your objectives:

- **Weight and Body Composition**: Track changes in weight, body fat percentage, and measurements (e.g., waist, hips, thighs).
- **Fitness Levels**: Measure improvements in cardiovascular endurance, strength (e.g., muscle strength and endurance), flexibility, and agility.

- **Nutritional Intake**: Monitor daily food intake, including calories, macronutrients (proteins, carbohydrates, fats), and micronutrients (vitamins, minerals).

Utilize Tracking Tools and Methods

Employ a variety of tools and methods to monitor your progress effectively:

- **Fitness Apps and Wearables**: Use apps or wearable devices to track workouts, steps taken, heart rate, and sleep patterns.
- **Measurement Tools**: Utilize scales, body composition analyzers, tape measures, and calipers to measure physical changes.
- **Fitness Assessments**: Conduct periodic assessments such as timed runs, strength tests, and flexibility assessments to gauge improvements.
- **Nutrition Logs**: Maintain food journals or use mobile apps to log meals, snacks, and beverages consumed throughout the day.

Regular Evaluation of Outcomes

Regularly assess your progress based on the tracked metrics and evaluations:

- **Compare against Goals**: Evaluate whether you are progressing towards your defined goals and objectives.

- **Adjust Strategies**: Identify areas where adjustments to your exercise routine, dietary habits, or lifestyle choices may be beneficial.
- **Celebrate Achievements**: Acknowledge and celebrate milestones and successes, reinforcing positive behaviors and motivation.

Tips for Effective Tracking

- **Consistency is Key**: Maintain consistent tracking habits to accurately monitor changes over time.
- **Be Honest and Accurate**: Record information truthfully to ensure reliable data for evaluation.
- **Review Periodically**: Schedule regular intervals (e.g., weekly, monthly) to review your progress and make adjustments as needed.

Adjusting Your Approach

Based on your evaluation of progress, make the necessary adjustments to optimize your journey:

- **Modify Goals**: Adjust timelines, set new milestones, or redefine specific targets based on your current progress and capabilities.
- **Adapt Strategies**: Modify workout routines, nutritional plans, or supplement regimens to better align with your evolving needs and preferences.
- **Seek Guidance**: Consult with fitness professionals, nutritionists, or healthcare providers for expert advice and support in refining your approach.

Tracking your progress provides valuable insights into your health and fitness journey, enabling you to make informed decisions and adjustments toward achieving your goals. By establishing clear metrics, utilizing effective tracking methods, regularly evaluating outcomes, and adjusting your approach as necessary, you can stay motivated, monitor your advancements, and navigate challenges effectively on the path to improved health and wellness. Remember to celebrate milestones and maintain a positive mindset as you work towards sustainable success in reaching your desired health outcomes.

6.2 Understanding Plateaus and How to Overcome Them

Plateaus are common in any health and fitness journey, where progress stalls despite continued efforts. Understanding why plateaus occur and employing effective strategies can help you overcome them and continue making advancements toward your goals.

What Causes Plateaus?

Plateaus can occur due to various reasons:

- **Adaptation**: The body adapts to repetitive workouts or dietary patterns, becoming more efficient and requiring different stimuli for continued progress.
- **Caloric Equilibrium**: Consuming the same amount of calories as you burn may halt weight loss or muscle gain.
- **Stress and Sleep**: Inadequate sleep or high-stress levels can affect hormone balance, metabolism, and recovery, impacting progress.

- **Nutrient Deficiencies**: Lack of essential nutrients or imbalanced diets can hinder performance and muscle growth.
- **Overtraining**: Excessive exercise without adequate recovery can lead to fatigue, decreased performance, and stalled progress.

Strategies to Overcome Plateaus

- **Evaluate and Adjust Goals**: Review your goals and consider adjusting timelines, targets, or strategies to stay motivated and focused.
- **Modify Exercise Routine**: Change workout intensity, frequency, duration, or type to challenge your body in new ways and prevent adaptation.
- **Dietary Adjustments**: Adjust caloric intake and macronutrient distribution based on current goals and energy needs. Ensure balanced nutrition to support performance and recovery.
- **Periodization**: Implement periodization principles in your training, alternating between phases of high intensity and recovery to optimize performance and prevent burnout.
- **Cross-Training**: Incorporate different types of exercises or activities (e.g., strength training, cardio, flexibility) to engage diverse muscle groups and stimulate overall fitness gains.
- **Rest and Recovery**: Prioritize adequate sleep and rest days to allow your body to repair, regenerate, and optimize performance.
- **Monitor Progress**: Continuously track your progress through measurements, fitness assessments, and performance metrics to identify trends and adjust strategies accordingly.
- **Seek Support**: Consult with fitness professionals, nutritionists, or healthcare providers for personalized guidance and advice tailored to your specific needs and challenges.

Mental Strategies

- **Stay Positive**: Maintain a positive mindset and focus on the progress you've made rather than solely on setbacks.
- **Stay Consistent**: Consistency is key to long-term success. Trust the process and remain committed to your health and fitness journey.
- **Celebrate Small Wins**: Acknowledge and celebrate every achievement, no matter how small, to reinforce positive behaviors and motivation.

Plateaus are a natural part of the health and fitness journey, but they can be overcome with proactive strategies and adjustments. By understanding the causes of plateaus, and implementing effective strategies such as modifying workouts, adjusting nutrition, prioritizing recovery, and seeking professional guidance, you can break through barriers and continue progressing toward your goals. Embrace challenges as opportunities for growth, stay persistent, and maintain a balanced approach to achieve sustainable success in your fitness journey.

6.3 Adapting Your Plan for Continued Success

Adapting your plan for continued success in your health and fitness journey involves making strategic adjustments to optimize progress, overcome challenges, and sustain long-term results. By proactively assessing your approach and implementing tailored modifications, you can maintain momentum and achieve your desired goals effectively.

Assess Current Progress

Begin by evaluating your current progress and outcomes:

- **Review Goals**: Assess whether you are on track to achieve your initial goals and objectives.
- **Measurements and Metrics**: Analyze measurements such as weight, body composition, fitness levels, and other relevant metrics tracked over time.
- **Performance Evaluation**: Evaluate improvements in strength, endurance, flexibility, and overall physical performance.

Identify Areas for Improvement

Identify specific areas where adjustments may be beneficial:

- **Plateau Identification**: Recognize any plateaus or stagnation in progress, where efforts have yielded diminishing returns.
- **Feedback and Observations**: Consider feedback from your body's response to exercise, nutrition, recovery, and overall lifestyle habits.

Strategies for Adaptation

Implement tailored strategies to adapt and optimize your plan:

1. Adjust Exercise Regimen:

Modify workout intensity, frequency, duration, and exercise selection to challenge your body and prevent adaptation.

Incorporate new exercises or training techniques to target different muscle groups and stimulate growth.

2. Revise Nutritional Approach:

Adjust caloric intake and macronutrient distribution based on current goals (e.g., weight loss, muscle gain).

Ensure adequate intake of essential nutrients to support performance, recovery, and overall health.

3. Enhance Recovery Practices:

Prioritize sufficient sleep and rest days to promote physical and mental recovery.

Incorporate relaxation techniques, such as yoga or meditation, to manage stress and enhance recovery.

4. Periodize Training:

Implement periodization principles, including cycles of varied intensity and volume, to optimize performance and prevent overtraining.

Schedule deload weeks or phases to facilitate recovery and prevent burnout.

5. Monitor and Adjust:

Continuously monitor progress through regular assessments and measurements.

Adjust strategies based on feedback, identifying what works best for your body and goals.

Seek Professional Guidance

Consult with fitness professionals, such as personal trainers or exercise physiologists, and healthcare providers, including registered dietitians or sports nutritionists, for expert advice and personalized recommendations:

- **Individualized Plans**: Receive tailored guidance and support to address specific challenges and optimize your plan for continued success.
- **Specialized Expertise**: Benefit from specialized knowledge and experience to navigate complexities related to training, nutrition, and overall health.

Stay Motivated and Consistent

Maintain motivation and consistency throughout your journey:

- **Set New Goals**: Establish realistic and challenging goals to maintain focus and drive.
- **Celebrate Achievements**: Acknowledge and celebrate milestones, no matter how small, to reinforce positive behaviors and maintain motivation.
- **Stay Flexible**: Embrace flexibility in your approach, adapting to changing circumstances or personal preferences while staying aligned with your overarching goals.

Adapting your plan for continued success involves a proactive approach to assessing progress, identifying areas for improvement, and implementing strategic adjustments. By evaluating current outcomes, identifying specific areas to optimize, and incorporating tailored strategies with professional guidance, you can sustain momentum, overcome challenges, and achieve sustainable results in your health and fitness journey. Stay committed, remain adaptable, and prioritize your well-being to foster long-term success and fulfillment in achieving your health and fitness goals.

6.4 Celebrating Milestones and Achievements

Celebrating milestones and achievements is crucial in maintaining motivation, reinforcing positive behaviors, and sustaining long-term success in your health and fitness journey. By acknowledging your progress and accomplishments, you not only boost confidence but also cultivate a positive mindset that fuels continued effort and dedication.

Importance of Celebrating Milestones

- **Motivation Boost**: Celebrating milestones provides a sense of accomplishment and motivation to keep progressing toward your goals.
- **Positive Reinforcement**: Recognition of achievements reinforces positive behaviors, making it more likely to continue healthy habits.
- **Reflection and Gratitude**: Reflecting on milestones encourages gratitude for progress made and inspires further dedication to your journey.

Types of Milestones to Celebrate

1. **Fitness Achievements:**

- Improvements in strength, endurance, flexibility, or overall fitness levels.
- Completing a challenging workout, achieving a personal best, or mastering a new exercise technique.

2. **Nutritional Milestones:**

- Consistently following a balanced nutrition plan or achieving dietary goals.

- Overcoming challenges like reducing sugar intake or increasing vegetable consumption.

3. Weight and Body Composition:

- Reaching a specific weight loss or muscle gain milestone.
- Decreasing body fat percentage or achieving a healthier body composition.

4. Lifestyle Changes:

- Adopting sustainable lifestyle habits such as regular exercise, adequate sleep, or stress management techniques.
- Making positive changes in overall well-being, such as improved mood, energy levels, or quality of life.

Ways to Celebrate Achievements

- **Set Rewards**: Establish rewards for reaching milestones, such as treating yourself to a favorite activity, buying new workout gear, or enjoying a healthy meal at a favorite restaurant.
- **Share Success**: Share your achievements with supportive friends, family members, or fitness communities to celebrate together and receive encouragement.
- **Create a Scrapbook or Journal**: Document your journey with photos, journal entries, or milestone markers to track progress and celebrate milestones visually.

- **Reflect and Appreciate**: Take time to reflect on your journey, acknowledging the effort and dedication that led to each milestone. Practice gratitude for the journey and the achievements made.
- **Plan Ahead**: Set new goals or milestones to continue challenging yourself and maintain momentum in your health and fitness journey.

Building a Positive Mindset

- **Focus on Progress**: Emphasize progress over perfection, recognizing that each milestone achieved contributes to your overall success.
- **Stay Inspired**: Draw inspiration from past achievements to tackle future challenges with confidence and determination.
- **Learn from Setbacks**: View setbacks as opportunities for growth and resilience, adjusting your approach while maintaining a positive outlook.

Celebrating milestones and achievements is an essential part of your health and fitness journey, fostering motivation, reinforcing positive behaviors, and cultivating a mindset of gratitude and perseverance. By recognizing and celebrating your progress, you not only enhance your journey's enjoyment but also strengthen your commitment to achieving long-term success in health and well-being. Embrace each milestone as a stepping stone towards your goals, and celebrate the journey as much as the destination.

Chapter 7: Long-Term Success and Maintenance

Achieving long-term success and maintaining your health and fitness goals requires commitment, consistency, and a sustainable approach. This chapter explores strategies and principles to help you establish lasting habits, navigate challenges, and sustain your achievements over time.

Establishing Sustainable Habits

- **Consistency**: Maintain regular exercise routines, balanced nutrition, and healthy lifestyle habits consistently over time.
- **Gradual Progress**: Focus on gradual, sustainable progress rather than quick fixes or extreme measures that are difficult to maintain.
- **Behavioral Changes**: Implement lasting behavioral changes, such as mindful eating, stress management, and adequate sleep, to support long-term health.

Navigating Challenges

- **Plateaus**: Recognize and overcome plateaus by adjusting workout routines, and nutrition plans, and seeking support from health professionals.
- **Setbacks**: Learn from setbacks as opportunities for growth, resilience, and reevaluating your approach to health and fitness.
- **Lifestyle Changes**: Adapt to life changes by modifying your fitness regimen and nutrition goals to accommodate new circumstances.

Strategies for Long-Term Success

- **Goal Setting**: Set realistic and achievable goals that are adaptable to your evolving needs and priorities.
- **Monitoring and Adjusting**: Continuously monitor progress, adjust goals, and modify strategies based on feedback and changes in circumstances.
- **Support System**: Surround yourself with a supportive network of friends, family, or fitness communities to stay motivated and accountable.

Maintenance Tips

- **Mindful Eating**: Practice mindful eating habits to maintain a balanced diet and prevent overeating.
- **Regular Exercise**: Incorporate varied workouts, including strength training, cardio, and flexibility exercises, to promote overall fitness and prevent monotony.
- **Self-Care**: Prioritize self-care activities such as adequate sleep, stress management techniques, and relaxation practices to support overall well-being.

Building Resilience

- **Positive Mindset**: Cultivate a positive mindset by celebrating achievements, learning from setbacks, and staying focused on long-term goals.

- **Adaptability**: Embrace flexibility in your approach to health and fitness, adjusting goals and strategies as needed to maintain motivation and progress.
- **Continuous Learning**: Stay informed about health and fitness trends, research, and best practices to make informed decisions and optimize your journey.

Achieving long-term success in health and fitness requires dedication, adaptability, and a commitment to sustainable habits. By establishing realistic goals, navigating challenges, implementing effective strategies, and prioritizing self-care and resilience, you can maintain your achievements and enjoy a lifelong journey of health and well-being. Embrace the process, celebrate milestones, and build a foundation for lasting success in your health and fitness endeavors.

7.1 Transitioning from Weight Loss to Maintenance

Transitioning from weight loss to maintenance is a critical phase in your health and fitness journey, marking a shift from focusing on losing weight to sustaining your achievements in a balanced and sustainable manner. This transition requires strategic adjustments in your approach to nutrition, exercise, and overall lifestyle to maintain your progress and prevent weight regain.

Establishing Sustainable Habits

- **Gradual Caloric Adjustment**: Gradually adjust your calorie intake to align with maintenance needs, considering your current weight, activity level, and metabolic rate.
- **Balanced Nutrition**: Continue emphasizing nutrient-dense foods, including lean proteins, whole grains, fruits, vegetables, and healthy fats, to support overall health and energy levels.
- **Mindful Eating**: Practice mindful eating techniques, such as listening to hunger cues, eating slowly, and avoiding distractions, to prevent overeating and promote satisfaction.

Maintaining Physical Activity

- **Regular Exercise Routine**: Maintain a consistent exercise regimen that includes a variety of activities such as cardiovascular workouts, strength training, and flexibility exercises.
- **Intensity and Duration**: Adjust exercise intensity and duration to support maintenance goals, focusing on maintaining muscle mass, cardiovascular fitness, and overall health.
- **Incorporate Active Lifestyle**: Incorporate physical activity into daily routines, such as walking, biking, or taking the stairs, to promote continuous movement and calorie expenditure.

Monitoring Progress and Adjustments

- **Regular Assessments**: Monitor your weight, body measurements, and fitness levels periodically to track progress and identify any changes that may require adjustments.

- **Nutritional Monitoring**: Continue tracking food intake and nutritional habits to ensure balanced nutrition and identify areas for improvement or modification.
- **Behavioral Changes**: Maintain healthy behaviors and lifestyle habits developed during the weight loss phase, such as adequate sleep, stress management, and hydration.

Strategies for Long-Term Success

- **Goal Setting**: Set realistic maintenance goals, such as maintaining current weight within a certain range or sustaining fitness achievements, to stay motivated and focused.
- **Adaptability**: Be flexible in adjusting your nutrition and exercise routines based on lifestyle changes, seasonal variations, or personal preferences to maintain consistency.
- **Support System**: Seek support from healthcare professionals, fitness trainers, or support groups to stay accountable, motivated, and informed about maintenance strategies.

Psychological and Emotional Well-Being

- **Celebrate Achievements**: Acknowledge and celebrate milestones reached during your weight loss journey to reinforce positive behaviors and maintain motivation.
- **Manage Stress**: Implement stress management techniques, such as meditation, yoga, or hobbies, to reduce stress levels that may impact eating habits and overall well-being.

- **Positive Mindset**: Cultivate a positive mindset by focusing on the benefits of maintaining a healthy weight and lifestyle, rather than solely on the number on the scale.

Transitioning from weight loss to maintenance requires a thoughtful and balanced approach that integrates sustainable habits, regular physical activity, monitoring progress, and maintaining emotional well-being. By establishing realistic goals, adapting your strategies as needed, and prioritizing long-term health and wellness, you can successfully navigate this phase of your journey and sustain your achievements for years to come. Embrace the journey of maintenance as an opportunity for continued growth, resilience, and lifelong well-being.

7.2 Maintaining a Healthy Lifestyle

Maintaining a healthy lifestyle is essential for long-term well-being and vitality. It involves adopting sustainable habits across nutrition, physical activity, stress management, and overall self-care to support optimal health and prevent chronic diseases. This chapter explores key principles and strategies for maintaining a healthy lifestyle beyond specific weight or fitness goals.

Balanced Nutrition

- **Nutrient-Dense Foods**: Emphasize a diet rich in fruits, vegetables, whole grains, lean proteins, and healthy fats to provide essential nutrients and promote overall health.

- **Portion Control**: Practice mindful eating and portion control to maintain a balanced caloric intake that aligns with your energy needs and promotes weight management.
- **Hydration**: Stay hydrated by consuming an adequate amount of water throughout the day, as hydration plays a crucial role in various bodily functions and overall well-being.

Regular Physical Activity

- **Consistent Exercise Routine**: Engage in regular physical activity, including aerobic exercises (e.g., walking, running, swimming), strength training, and flexibility exercises, to promote cardiovascular health, muscular strength, and flexibility.
- **Daily Movement**: Incorporate physical activity into daily routines, such as taking walks, using stairs instead of elevators, or participating in active hobbies, to maintain an active lifestyle.
- **Variety and Enjoyment**: Choose activities that you enjoy and vary your workouts to prevent boredom, maintain motivation, and engage different muscle groups.

Stress Management

- **Stress Reduction Techniques**: Practice stress management techniques such as deep breathing, meditation, yoga, or spending time in nature to reduce stress levels and promote relaxation.
- **Work-Life Balance**: Maintain a healthy balance between work, personal life, and leisure activities to minimize stress and enhance overall well-being.

- **Quality Sleep**: Prioritize adequate sleep (7-9 hours per night for adults) to support physical and mental health, promote recovery, and enhance daytime productivity.

Preventive Health Practices

- **Regular Health Check-ups**: Schedule regular health screenings and check-ups with healthcare professionals to monitor your overall health status and detect any potential health issues early.
- **Healthy Relationships**: Cultivate supportive relationships with friends, family, and community members to enhance emotional well-being and social support.
- **Avoidance of Harmful Substances**: Minimize or avoid the use of harmful substances such as tobacco, excessive alcohol, and illicit drugs to protect overall health and well-being.

Lifelong Learning and Growth

- **Continuous Education**: Stay informed about health and wellness topics, advancements in nutrition and fitness, and evidence-based practices to make informed decisions about your health.
- **Adaptability**: Be open to adjusting your habits, goals, and routines as life circumstances change to maintain consistency and sustainability in your healthy lifestyle.
- **Positive Mindset**: Foster a positive outlook on life by practicing gratitude, setting realistic goals, celebrating achievements, and embracing challenges as opportunities for growth.

Maintaining a healthy lifestyle involves integrating sustainable habits across nutrition, physical activity, stress management, and overall well-being. By prioritizing balanced nutrition, regular physical activity, effective stress management, preventive health practices, continuous learning, and a positive mindset, you can enhance your quality of life, reduce the risk of chronic diseases, and promote long-term well-being. Embrace these principles as a foundation for lifelong health and vitality, adapting and refining your approach to support your evolving health goals and needs.

7.3 Dealing with Setbacks and Relapses

Dealing with setbacks and relapses is a natural part of any health and wellness journey. Whether it's a temporary lapse in healthy habits or a significant challenge that interrupts your progress, learning to effectively manage setbacks is crucial for maintaining long-term success and resilience. This chapter explores strategies and techniques to navigate setbacks and relapses effectively.

Understanding Setbacks

1. **Common Causes:**

- **Stress and Emotional Triggers**: Emotional stress, life changes, or challenging situations can lead to lapses in healthy behaviors.
- **Lack of Planning**: Inadequate preparation or changes in routine may disrupt healthy habits like meal planning or exercise.

- **Social and Environmental Influences**: Social events, peer pressure, or environments unsupportive of healthy choices can contribute to setbacks.

Types of Setbacks:

- **Minor Lapses**: Short-term deviations from healthy habits, such as skipping workouts or indulging in unhealthy foods occasionally.
- **Major Challenges**: Significant setbacks, such as returning to old habits for an extended period or experiencing a decline in overall well-being.

Strategies for Managing Setbacks

1. **Self-Compassion and Acceptance:**

- Practice self-compassion by acknowledging setbacks as part of the journey and avoiding self-blame or guilt.
- Accept the situation without judgment, recognizing that setbacks provide opportunities for growth and learning.

2. **Identify Triggers and Patterns:**

- Reflect on triggers or situations that led to the setback, such as stress, boredom, or social influences.

- Identify patterns in behavior or thought processes that may contribute to lapses in healthy habits.

3. Develop Coping Strategies:

- Build a toolkit of coping strategies, such as deep breathing, mindfulness exercises, or talking to a supportive friend or mentor, to manage stress and emotional triggers effectively.
- Engage in activities that promote relaxation and emotional well-being, such as meditation, yoga, or spending time in nature.

4. Reassess Goals and Priorities:

- Review your health and wellness goals to ensure they are realistic and aligned with your current priorities and circumstances.
- Adjust goals or timelines as needed to accommodate setbacks or changes in your journey.

Getting Back on Track

1. Set Specific and Attainable Goals:

- Set small, achievable goals to regain momentum and rebuild confidence in your ability to make healthy choices.
- Break larger goals into manageable steps to facilitate progress and maintain motivation.

2. Resume Healthy Habits Gradually:

- Start reintroducing healthy habits gradually, focusing on consistency rather than perfection.
- Prioritize foundational habits such as nutritious eating, regular exercise, and adequate sleep to support overall well-being.

3. Seek Support and Accountability:

- Reach out to a supportive network of friends, family, or a health professional for encouragement, guidance, and accountability.
- Consider joining a support group, or fitness class, or seeking the guidance of a coach or counselor specializing in behavior change.

Learning from Setbacks

1. Reflect and Learn:

- Reflect on the experience and lessons learned from setbacks to identify areas for personal growth and improvement.
- Use setbacks as opportunities to strengthen resilience, develop new coping strategies, and refine your approach to achieving long-term health and wellness.

2. Stay Positive and Persistent:

- Maintain a positive mindset by focusing on progress made and celebrating small victories along the way.
- Stay persistent in your commitment to health and wellness, recognizing that setbacks are temporary and part of the journey toward lasting change.

Dealing with setbacks and relapses requires patience, self-compassion, and a proactive approach to managing challenges effectively. By understanding the causes of setbacks, developing coping strategies, reassessing goals, and seeking support when needed, you can navigate setbacks with resilience and continue progressing toward your health and wellness goals. Embrace setbacks as opportunities for growth, learn from the experience, and stay committed to building a healthy lifestyle that supports your overall well-being and long-term success.

7.4 Building a Support System

Building a support system is essential for maintaining motivation, accountability, and resilience on your health and wellness journey. A strong support system provides encouragement, guidance, and practical assistance during both triumphs and challenges. Here's how to cultivate a supportive network to enhance your success in adopting and maintaining a healthy lifestyle.

Firstly, identify individuals in your life who can contribute positively to your journey. This may include close friends, family members, coworkers, or mentors who share similar health goals or are supportive of your aspirations. Communicate openly with them about your goals, challenges, and progress, fostering an environment of trust and mutual support.

Secondly, seek out structured support networks such as fitness groups, exercise classes, or online communities focused on health and wellness. These communities can offer camaraderie, shared experiences, and valuable insights from individuals facing similar challenges.

Thirdly, consider professional support from healthcare providers, nutritionists, personal trainers, or counselors specializing in behavior change. These professionals can provide expert guidance, personalized strategies, and evidence-based recommendations to optimize your health journey.

Additionally, engage in reciprocal support by offering encouragement and assistance to others pursuing their health goals. By contributing positively to someone else's journey, you can strengthen your commitment, gain perspective, and foster meaningful connections within your support system.

Finally, maintain regular communication and engagement with your support network. Share successes, seek advice during setbacks, and celebrate milestones together. Utilize various communication channels such as in-person meetings, phone calls, social media groups, or virtual platforms to stay connected and motivated.

In conclusion, building a support system is a vital component of sustaining motivation, accountability, and resilience in your pursuit of a healthy lifestyle. By cultivating relationships with supportive individuals, participating in structured communities, seeking professional guidance, offering reciprocal support, and maintaining open communication, you can enhance your ability to achieve and maintain long-term health and wellness goals. Embrace the power of a supportive network to navigate challenges, celebrate successes, and enjoy the journey towards a healthier, happier life.

7.5 The Journey to Lifelong Health and Fitness

The journey to lifelong health and fitness is a continuous pursuit of well-being, vitality, and overall quality of life. It transcends short-term goals and embraces a holistic approach to physical, mental, and emotional wellness. This chapter explores key principles and strategies to foster sustainable habits, maintain motivation, and achieve lasting health and fitness.

Embracing Sustainable Habits

- **Balanced Nutrition**: Prioritize a balanced diet rich in nutrient-dense foods such as fruits, vegetables, whole grains, lean proteins, and healthy fats. Adopt mindful eating practices to support nutritional needs and promote satiety.
- **Regular Physical Activity**: Engage in regular exercise routines that incorporate cardiovascular workouts, strength training, flexibility exercises, and recreational activities. Aim for consistency and variety to enhance overall fitness and prevent monotony.
- **Stress Management**: Implement stress reduction techniques such as meditation, deep breathing, yoga, or spending time in nature. Prioritize self-care activities to promote relaxation and mental well-being.

Cultivating a Positive Mindset

- **Goal Setting**: Set realistic and achievable goals that align with your values and priorities. Break larger goals into smaller milestones to track progress and maintain motivation.
- **Self-Compassion**: Practice self-compassion and acceptance during setbacks or challenges. Learn from experiences, adjust strategies as needed, and celebrate successes along the way.
- **Resilience**: Build resilience by adapting to changes, learning from failures, and maintaining a positive outlook. Embrace challenges as opportunities for growth and personal development.

Seeking Support and Accountability

- **Building a Support System**: Surround yourself with a supportive network of friends, family, mentors, or health professionals who encourage and inspire your journey. Share successes, seek guidance during setbacks, and celebrate achievements together.
- **Professional Guidance**: Consult with healthcare providers, nutritionists, personal trainers, or counselors to receive expert advice, personalized strategies, and evidence-based recommendations for optimizing your health and fitness journey.

Lifelong Learning and Adaptability

- **Continuous Education**: Stay informed about current health trends, scientific research, and best practices in nutrition, exercise science, and wellness. Seek opportunities for learning and personal growth to refine your approach over time.
- **Adaptability**: Remain flexible in adjusting your goals, strategies, and routines based on changing circumstances, lifestyle

preferences, or new insights. Embrace a dynamic approach that evolves with your journey toward lifelong health.

Celebrating the Journey

- **Gratitude**: Cultivate gratitude for your body's capabilities, achievements, and the support system that empowers your progress. Reflect on how far you've come and acknowledge the efforts invested in your health and well-being.
- **Enjoyment**: Find joy in the process of pursuing health and fitness goals. Engage in activities you love, explore new challenges, and prioritize activities that contribute positively to your overall well-being.

The journey to lifelong health and fitness is a transformative path that requires dedication, resilience, and a commitment to sustainable habits. By embracing balanced nutrition, regular physical activity, stress management techniques, cultivating a positive mindset, seeking support, and adapting to life's changes, you can achieve lasting health and fitness. Embrace the journey as an opportunity for growth, self-discovery, and the pursuit of a vibrant, fulfilling life. Stay motivated, stay committed, and enjoy the rewards of a lifelong commitment to your health and well-being.

Conclusion:

In this comprehensive guide to weight loss for women, we've explored proven strategies and techniques designed to empower you on your journey toward achieving health and fitness goals. Throughout this book, we've delved into the science of weight loss, debunked common myths, and provided practical advice on nutrition, exercise, and lifestyle adjustments tailored specifically for women.

Achieving sustainable weight loss involves more than just shedding pounds—it's about adopting lifelong habits that support overall well-being and vitality. By focusing on balanced nutrition, regular physical activity, stress management, and building a supportive network, you can transform your body and enhance your quality of life.

Key Takeaways:

- **Understanding Your Body**: Recognize the unique factors influencing weight loss for women, including metabolic differences, hormonal fluctuations, and lifestyle habits.
- **Nutrition Essentials**: Embrace a balanced diet rich in whole foods, lean proteins, fruits, vegetables, and healthy fats. Practice mindful eating and portion control to support weight management and overall health.
- **Effective Exercise Strategies**: Incorporate a variety of workouts that include cardio, strength training, flexibility exercises, and active living to improve fitness levels and maintain muscle mass.
- **Lifestyle and Behavioral Changes**: Build healthy habits such as adequate sleep, stress management techniques, and strategies for overcoming emotional eating to sustain long-term success.

- **Monitoring Progress and Adjusting Goals**: Track your progress, celebrate achievements, and reassess goals regularly to stay motivated and adaptable to changes in your journey.
- **Building a Support System**: Surround yourself with supportive individuals who encourage and inspire your efforts toward health and fitness. Seek professional guidance and community support to enhance accountability and motivation.

As you continue on your path to wellness, remember that each step forward is a testament to your dedication and resilience. Embrace setbacks as learning opportunities, practice self-compassion, and celebrate every milestone achieved along the way.

By integrating the knowledge and strategies from this guide into your daily life, you have the power to transform your body, elevate your health, and achieve your fitness goals. Your journey towards weight loss and lifelong well-being is a testament to your strength and commitment—embrace it, enjoy it, and thrive in the healthier, happier version of yourself.

Here's to your success in achieving and maintaining a vibrant, balanced lifestyle. Keep moving forward, one positive choice at a time.

Stay healthy. Stay motivated. Stay empowered.